TOTAL QUALITY MANAGEMENT IN HEALTHCARE

Implementation Strategies for Optimum Results

D. H. Stamatis

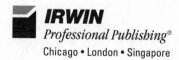

IRWIN
Professional Publishing®
Chicago • London • Singapore

Times Mirror
Higher Education Group

Library of Congress Cataloging-in-Publication Data

Stamatis, D. H.
   Total quality management in healthcare : implementation strategies for optimum results / D.H. Stamatis.
      p.   cm.
   ISBN 0-7863-0980-6
   "A Healthcare 2000 publication."
   Includes index.
   1. Medical care—Quality control.   2. Total quality management.   3. Health services administration.
RA399.A1 S73   1996
362.1/068/5—dc20   96-01634

Printed in the United States of America
1 2 3 4 5 6 7 8 9 0 BS 3 2 1 0 9 8 7 6

In memory of
Taki

Over the last 10 years the world of manufacturing has been exposed to a revolutionary philosophy called Total Quality Management (TQM). Great improvements have been associated with its introduction, and everyone—at least it seems that way—has positive things to say about it.

A lot has been written about this TQM as it applies to manufacturing. However, it is indeed a late development to talk about TQM healthcare. In my last book, *Total Quality Service*, we addressed the general concerns about quality as it relates to service. We discussed the general concepts of service quality, the tools used, and three separate models for implementation. Furthermore, we gave many examples of both concepts and real situations.

In this book, we are going to be very specific about quality in healthcare, since quality *works not only in manufacturing but also in services, hospitals, government, and even schools*. It is a revolution in everything we do. We are going to approach this revolution from a point of view that will identify areas of decreased costs, fewer mistakes, less rework, happier workers, and delighted customers.

The focus of the book is to synthesize the generally accepted philosophies of quality—Juran, Crosby, Taguchi, and Deming—and to provide a model for the implementation process as well as the specific tools that will identify, measure, and evaluate the quality efforts in the organization. Our emphasis will be on the following:

1. Why the foremost purpose of business and each employee is to understand and satisfy the requirements of internal and external customers.
2. How employee performance is greatly enhanced by worker empowerment.
3. Why to bother with continuous improvement.
4. What management excellence has to do with TQM.

The audience of the book is designed to be both management and nonmanagement personnel who work in healthcare. They may have some background in TQM, or they may be totally new to the philosophy. In either case, the book is designed to be self-contained and each of its chapters to be independent of each other. The reader may choose to "jump around" depending on the information he or she is seeking.

ACKNOWLEDGMENTS

No book is ever the product of one individual. This book is no different. I owe a lot to many individuals who have helped either in a direct or in an indirect way and have made possible this book.

Special thanks go to the Hospital Corporation of America, HCA Management Company (now Columbia Healthcare), and Henry Ford Hospital Educational Training Services for granting me permission to use the figures dealing with the Quality Improvement Roadmap.

I want to thank my most precious advisor and editor, Carla, not only for her support but also for the insightful information that she provided throughout the project. Her critical care nursing background has proven very beneficial.

I want to thank Mr. J. Stewart from St. Claire Hospital for his lengthy discussions on the issues of healthcare and on the issues of management and the leadership role as they effect modern day healthcare. I have tried to incorporate his wisdom as much as possible.

I want to thank Mr. R. Stark from St. Claire Hospital for his support, suggestions, and recommendations in the area of team dynamics.

I want to thank Mr. M. S. Meiss from the Oakwood Hospital and Medical Center for his suggestions and recommendations.

I want to thank Dr. D. Carey from Henry Ford Hospital for his valuable suggestions.

I also want to thank Drs. G. Bletsas, R. R. Yalamanchi, and S. R. Kaura for their suggestions from their self-employed perspective.

I want to thank Drs. G. Dounis and K. Dounis from the Veteran's Administration Hospital.

I want to thank Mr. J. Kontos from Henry Ford Hospital for his suggestions and recommendations throughout the project.

I want to thank the staff of North Central Bronx Hospital for their patience and recommendations in addressing the tools of TQM.

I also want to thank Ms. S. A. Gorecki, a student at Central Michigan University, for her suggestions after reading earlier drafts.

I want to thank Dr. D. Pallas from Henry Ford Hospital for his thought provoking and very valuable suggestions.

I also want to thank Miss D. Sengos from Harper-Grace Hospital for her comments and suggestions as well as encouragement throughout the project.

And I want to thank the editors at Irwin Professional Publishing for their support, editing, and very thoughtful suggestions throughout the project.

Finally, I want to thank all my seminar participants over the years for their questions, concerns, suggestions, and recommendations. I have tried to incorporate as many as possible.

Diomidis H. Stamatis

CONTENTS

Chapter 2

Overview of Total Quality Management in Healthcare   51

Chapter 3

Teams   65

Chapter 4

Data Collection and Analysis   87

Chapter 7

Advanced Topics of Quality   141

Chapter 8

ISO 9000 Standards and Healthcare   167

Chapter 9

Malcolm Baldrige National Quality Award and Healthcare   175

Chapter 10

Marketing System Design   197

PART TWO

DEPLOYMENT OF TQM   209

Chapter 11

How to Implement Total Quality Management   211

Chapter 12

Breakthrough Process   219

Chapter 13

A Case Study in Quality Management   271

Appendix D

TRAINING FOR BREAKTHROUGH STRATEGY IN HEALTHCARE   299

Appendix E

LESSONS LEARNED   303

Appendix F

FORMULAS USED IN QUALITY MANAGEMENT   307

Appendix G

CONTROL CHARTS   321

GLOSSARY   329

SELECTED BIBLIOGRAPHY   337

INDEX   343

LIST OF TABLES

LIST OF FIGURES

Why Total Quality Management?

It takes more than the latest technology to stay competitive in today's global marketplace. The skills, knowledge, and productivity of people as well as quality are still key to every organization's success.

Quality must be viewed as a *customer* determination. Quality is neither a marketing determination nor a management determination. It is based on customers' actual experience with the product or service, measured against their requirements—stated or unstated, conscious or sensed, technically operational or entirely subjective. Quality always represents a moving target in a competitive market.

THE NEED FOR QUALITY CONCEPTS

The old adage "An ounce of prevention is better than a pound of cure" is as appropriate to the industrial problem of unnecessary costs as it is to the medical problem of disease; if the causes for a problem can be analyzed and thereby understood, measures can be taken to prevent it from happening.

We have the techniques required to pursue such quality concepts, and they are covered under the umbrella of total quality management (TQM). Some of these specific techniques are advanced quality planning, statistical process control (SPC), design of experiments (DOE), quality of work life (QWL), quality circles, participative management programs, empowerment, self-directed teams, and quality function deployment (QFD). These techniques have been heralded as miracle measures because they are curing all sorts of problems across many industries, including healthcare. These problems have been recognized and labeled as unnecessary costs. Frequent euphemisms for these costs are errors, customer dissatisfaction, scrap, reject, rework, and warranty.

These unnecessary costs arise for various reasons, which are not at first readily apparent, especially to those individuals most responsible for causing them. The main causes, or reasons, may be classified into four main groups and a number of subgroups. The classification is listed as follows:

Causes of Unnecessary Costs
  A. Management inefficiency
      1. No commitment or ambivalent commitment
      2. Lack of competency
      3. Lack of a vision for quality, that is, objectives
      4. Lack of planning
      5. Lack of pressure
      6. Lack of training
  B. Inability to apply quality consideration
      1. Lack of information
      2. Lack of communication
      3. Lack of ideas
  C. Competitive pressures
      1. Lack of time
  D. Human weaknesses
      1. Honest wrong beliefs
      2. Habits and attitudes
      3. Gold plating (always sugarcoating problems) or playing it safe
      4. Pride

It is worth noting that most of the causes are due to the *lack* of something, which in most cases, reasonably well-organized companies can provide without a great deal of difficulty. The human weaknesses referred to are nearly always present in all known endeavors, and their understanding is beneficial apart from the role they play in the search for total quality.

THE HEALTHCARE ENVIRONMENT

Within healthcare, problems are being generated faster than we can address them. This problem is expected to continue into the 21st century. In the United States, healthcare costs have been escalating for the past 30 years. In 1960 annual healthcare expenditures for the entire country were $27.1 billion. In 1990 those expenditures rose to $666.2 billion, and just two years later annual health expenditures were more than $900 billion. By the year 2000 it is estimated that the price of healthcare for our nation will reach $1.9 trillion, if the same percentage of growth continues as in the 1980s and 1990s (Bryja et al. 1992).

Obviously, something has to be done about the rise in healthcare costs, which is occurring too fast for the economy and the nation to bear. There have been many suggestions to correct the problem, including TQM, managed care, managed competition, healthcare mergers, international healthcare consortiums, alternative medicine, domestic healthcare alliances, third-party control (redesigned health insurance products) through health maintenance organizations (HMOs) or independent administrators. Additionally, individual co-payments, reduction of healthcare as a fringe benefit, and a freeze in doctors' fees, etc., have been suggested to improve the efficiency of access to care and to minimize costs in healthcare. This book will discuss only the issue of total quality management as it relates to healthcare.

Why TQM? Because it provides four essential principles for healthcare reform, which is needed today and in the future. These principles are:

1. Measure quality, so that you can manage it.
2. Focus on the patient, so that you may satisfy him or her.
3. Tap the brainpower of everyone in the organization, so that you may take advantage of synergy.
4. Plan strategically, so that you may think long term but act in the short term.

In essence, TQM becomes the hinge for understanding and improving both the inward and outward focus of the organization. It does that by systematically formulating and communicating that focus to both internal and external customers.

POLITICAL PERSPECTIVES AND PRESSURES

All players in the political arena (both national and state politicians) have proposed major changes in healthcare, primarily because they say that healthcare is in crisis. Part of that crisis is in the area of quality with its many definitions. The changes openly discussed in the media over the last three years will be in all areas of healthcare. Although the scope of this book is not to be political or to address any specifics, it would be unfair to the reader if we did not at least summarize some of the points that the plans suggest collectively. The summary that follows is by no means comprehensive. If one was to summarize the plans in their entirety and extract the foundations for the proposed changes, two points become obvious and of paramount importance. They are:

1. If change is to occur, all health plans must operate in a highly regulated environment.
2. Within this regulated environment, there must be a great deal of flexibility among the states.

In addition to these two points, in the national forum of discussion there has been a movement to discuss healthcare from several points of view. Of course, as of this writing, none of them have materialized; however, the discussion continues. Some of the predominant points of view discussed are access to care, structure of the healthcare system, healthcare benefits, cost containment, financing of healthcare, and malpractice reform.

Access to Care

Under a proposal for a national healthcare system, all citizens would be guaranteed health insurance coverage with a standardized benefit package and would receive coverage through a health alliance. All individuals would be required to enroll in a health plan. During the transitional period, to be defined at some future time, the Secretary of Health and Human Services (HHS) would be authorized to establish a national risk pool to make health insurance available to the uninsured. Enrollment would be voluntary. Assessments would be imposed on all insurers to support the program.

Employers would be required to pay a percentage of the average weighted premium for the alliance. Employees would be required to pay the remainder of the premium for the health plan they select. Subsidies would be available for certain low-wage employers and employees. All employers would be required to contribute to their employees' healthcare. Employers with fewer than 5,000 employees would operate through the regional alliances. Employers with greater than 5,000 employees can form corporate alliances and bypass the regional alliance system.

Structure of the Healthcare System

National Health Board
A national health board has been discussed, to be the central body of authority that enforces all health policies. This board may be at a state or national level. The board would approve state plans for implementing reform through health alliances or a single payer system. It would set the formula for risk adjusters for use in calculation of payments to health plans.

Health Alliances
Another proposal is that each state must establish one or more regional health alliances. An alliance may not cross state lines, but two or more contiguous states may coordinate the operation of alliances.

Everyone, with the following exceptions, would get health insurance coverage through some form of alliance. The Federal Employee Health Benefits Pension (FEHBP) and Medicaid would be brought into the alliance system. Medicare will remain separate, unless a state chooses to bring Medicare beneficiaries into the system. The Department of Veterans Affairs (VA), and the Indian Health Service may gradually be integrated into the system.

Alliances would contract with health plans that meet state standards. Each alliance must offer one fee-for-service plan that must operate under a budget. The fee-for-service plan would negotiate a fee schedule with the alliance and would monitor its physicians with respect to the budget and utilization. The plan could reduce payments to providers as necessary to keep costs within budget.

Health Plans

Health plans must meet uniform conditions of participation in a health alliance including those related to the following:

- Truth in marketing.
- Fiscal soundness.
- Verifying credentials of providers and facilities.
- Consumer protection.
- Confidentiality.
- Complaint procedures.
- Disenrollment for cause.
- Utilization management.
- Data management and reporting.

There also must be provisions for reimbursement. All plans must participate in a guarantee fund. If a health plan fails, states may assess payments of a certain percentage as a premium, on other health plans within the alliance, to generate revenue to cover outstanding claims.

State Flexibility

States would be responsible for setting the standards (solvency, data collection, quality assurance, etc.) that health plans must meet to participate in the system. States do not set structural requirements for health plans (i.e., provider organizations). States would establish the mechanisms for the governance of health alliances as well as the geographic boundaries of alliances. Finally, a state may establish a single-payer healthcare system.

Healthcare Benefits

All health plans would be required to offer a standardized health benefit package, initially set in stature and then updated by the National Health Board, which would emphasize primary and preventive services. The plans would offer three choices of cost sharing:

- *Low cost sharing*. Health plan members would make nominal payments (e.g., a low fee for outpatient services, no copayment for inpatient services), but there would be a 40% coinsurance for optional point-of-service offering.

- *Higher cost sharing.* Participants would pay deductibles of specified amounts.
- *Combination.* Participants would have low cost sharing if they used preferred providers and higher cost sharing if they used out-of-network providers.

Cost Containment

Short-term cost containment would not be mandatory. However, there would be future limits on Medicare and Medicaid spending. For the private sector, there would not be a cap on an individual plan's premium increases.

Financing of Healthcare

The following sources of healthcare financing have been proposed:

- Increased taxes on packs of cigarettes and on hard liquor.
- Medicare and Medicaid savings.
- Revenues anticipated from income taxes attributable to employer savings from lower healthcare costs.
- Other unspecified federal savings.

Malpractice Reform

The development and adoption of alternative dispute resolution mechanisms (e.g., arbitration or mediation) make up the centerpiece of the malpractice reform proposal. States could use federal funds to establish enterprise liability demonstration projects to determine the value of substituting health plan liability for physician liability.

JOINT COMMISSION

The Joint Commission on Accreditation of Healthcare Organizations (JCAHO) is an organization that tries to define and improve healthcare practices by evaluating and accrediting healthcare organizations. It has been doing it for a long time, and one of its major accomplishments is that over the years it has been able to identify, track, and measure key characteristics in healthcare. It is beyond the scope of this book to address the Joint Commission's agenda and practices. However, if the reader is interested in more details about JCAHO accreditation methods and rationale, I refer them to the Joint Commission's *1995 Comprehensive Accreditation Manual for Hospitals* (1994).

The principles embodied in the JCAHO may be summarized in the following:

- Standards should emphasize actual organizational performance, not simply the capacity to perform.
- Standards should address what counts: the care provided to the patient and the management of the organization. These are what make the difference in quality for the patient.
- In these broad areas of patient care and management, standards should focus on important activities, or functions, that significantly influence, directly or indirectly, eventual patient outcomes. Simply stated, hospitals should be doing the right things and doing them well.
- The performance expectations reflected in the standards should be set forth in a quality improvement context. The objective is not to punish competent practitioners and staff but rather to improve the internal systems and work environment that help them and their organization realize their primary goal. That goal is excellent care which continues to improve over time.

How is the JCAHO trying to accomplish this ambition? By having identified four critical areas in the delivery process of high-quality healthcare. These four areas are:

1. Leadership
   a. Develop a mission
   b. Develop a vision
   c. Develop priorities
   d. Develop resources
2. Management of human resources
   a. Education
   b. Competence
3. Management of information
   a. Planning
   b. Aggregate data

    c. Comparative data
    d. Knowledge-based data
  4. Improvement of organizational performance
    a. Collaboration
    b. Process thinking

These major areas are broken down into three categories: patient-focused functions, organizational functions, and structures with functions. Each of the categories is subdivided even further and assigned a numerical score during the Joint Commission's review process. The specific categories on which organizations are critiqued are:

  I. Patient-Focused Functions
    A. Patient rights and organizational ethics
      1. Patient rights
      2. Organizational ethics
    B. Assessment of patients
      1. Initial assessment
      2. Pathology and clinical laboratory
      3. Reassessment
      4. Care decisions
      5. Structures supporting the assessment of patients
      6. Additional requirements for specific patient populations
    C. Care of patients
      1. Planning and providing care
      2. Anesthesia care
      3. Medication care
      4. Operative and other invasive procedures
      5. Rehabilitation care and services
      6. Special treatment procedures
    D. Education
      1. Patient and family education and responsibilities
    E. Continuum of care
      1. Consistency in quality care
  II. Organizational Functions
    A. Improving organizational performance
      1. Plan
      2. Design
      3. Measure

      4. Assess
      5. Improve
   B. Leadership
      1. Organizational planning
      2. Directing departments
      3. Integrating services
      4. Role in improving performance
   C. Management of the environment of care
      1. Design
      2. Implementation
      3. Measurement systems
      4. Social environment
   D. Management of human resources
      1. Human resources planning
      2. Organization, training, and education of staff
      3. Competence assessment
      4. Staff rights mechanisms
   E. Management of information
      1. Information management planning
      2. Patient-specific data and information
      3. Aggregate data and information
      4. Knowledge-based information
      5. Comparative data and information
   F. Surveillance, prevention, and control of infection
III. Structures with Functions
   A. Governance
      1. The style we govern
   B. Management
      1. The style we manage
   C. Medical staff
      1. Organization, bylaws, and rules and regulations
      2. Credentialing
   D. Nursing
      1. Nursing policies and procedures
      2. Standards of nursing practice

For each category, the JCAHO survey team assigns a score, with 1 signifying substantial compliance and 5 signifying no compliance. N and P signify not applicable and primary service, respectively.

Accreditation Decisions

The Joint Commission makes five types of accreditation decisions.

Accreditation with commendation: This is the highest accreditation decision, awarded to an organization that has demonstrated exemplary performance.

Accreditation: This decision indicates that an organization is in overall compliance with applicable standards. Accreditation is awarded either with or without type 1 recommendations. A type 1 recommendation is a recommendation or a group of recommendations that must be resolved within a specified period of time or the organization risks losing its accreditation.

Provisional accreditation: This is an accreditation decision that results when an organization has demonstrated substantial compliance with the selected structural standards surveyed in the first of two surveys conducted under the Early Survey Policy. The second survey is conducted approximately six months later to allow the organization sufficient time to demonstrate a track record of performance. Provisional accreditation status remains until the organization completes this second, full survey.

Conditional accreditation: This decision indicates that multiple and substantial deficiencies in compliance with the standards exist in an organization. Correction of deficiencies serves as the basis for further consideration of continuing accreditation and must be demonstrated through a follow-up survey.

Not accredited: This accreditation decision results when an organization has been denied accreditation, when its accreditation is withdrawn by the Joint Commission, or when it withdraws from the accreditation process. This designation also describes any organization that has never applied for accreditation.

JCAHO versus TQM Efforts

One can see that the JCAHO is making great strides to implement quality systems in healthcare. There are many good aspects of quality built into the system, for example, prevention, continual improvement, and management. However, it still falls short on defining customer satisfaction and providing guidance on the use of statistical thinking for the process. The strict definition of the patient as a customer is very limited. It should be expanded to cover "the next person" or the "next process." The same holds true for the definition of "process." It should be expanded and redefined because unless it is, the section on management of information is going to generate limited, biased, and incomplete information.

The JCAHO is doing an excellent job in identifying shortcomings of organizations, but much more may be done through a TQM implementation in the same organizations. Table 1 shows a cursory view of the Joint Commission's approach and TQM's approach to quality in healthcare. A full discussion of TQM implementation will be addressed in Chapter 11.

COMMENTS ON MANAGED CARE

As important as healthcare is, it is amazing that none of the political figures or members of the beltway media and think-tank organizations are addressing healthcare reform from a quality perspective. They all have figured out that reform is imminent but are going about it in all directions. They want to change one bureaucratic system for another, without the new knowledge that we have about quality management. The notions of prevention as opposed to appraisal, such as cost of quality, empowerment, reengineering, teams, and statistical process control, to name a few, have completely eluded all of them. No one at any level of government is talking about things that actually can bring healthcare costs under control.

An example of the mumbo jumbo jargon is the managed care controversy. Will managed medical care be hazardous to your health? Will the cost-cutting forces of the marketplace overwhelm traditional medical morality and put the United States at risk of losing the best healthcare the world has ever known? I categorically believe so. The reason for such belief is that the healthcare system is moving quickly in imposing profit-driven systems of medical care on both physicians and patients. Unfortunately, profitability is the name of the game, as opposed to improving the health system.

As Dr. J. Kassirer, editor-in-chief of the *New England Journal of Medicine,* has observed (Beck 1995), market-driven care is likely to alienate physicians, undermine patients' trust of physicians' motives, cripple academic medical centers, handicap the research es-

T A B L E   1

Comparison of JCAHO's 10 Steps and TQM

JCAHO's Steps	How TQM Can Help
1. Assign responsibility	Provides reports to the board of trustees, administration, and medical staff to monitor and evaluate clinical activities
2. Delineate scope of care	Assesses clinical performance by service
3. Identify important aspects of care	Identifies key functions, treatments, activities, and outcomes
4. Identify indicators	Includes a benchmarking approach of other similar medical facilities to establish objective and measurable indicators
5. Establish thresholds for evaluation	Establishes statistically significant thresholds by comparing indicators across national or customized norms through benchmarking
6. Collect and organize data	Uses existing data and organizes it into standard reports
7. Evaluate care when thresholds are reached	Identifies statistically meaningful areas of exemplary performance and opportunities for quality improvement; provides individual patient listings for focused review
8. Take actions to improve care	Identifies processes of care for corrective action
9. Assess effectiveness and maintain the gain	Continuously monitors all indicators to document changes in performance over time
10. Communicate results	Provides standardized, trend, and executive reports for clear examples of effective quality improvement and aids in communicating key issues

tablishment, and expand the population of patients who have no healthcare insurance. Another example of market-driven care is the capitated system in which patients (or their employers or insurers) pay a fixed amount regardless of how much care they receive and the plan has a financial incentive to spend as little as possible of that care. Physicians in such systems may have their earnings cut if they prescribe too much costly treatment. So why should they? The incentive to remain employed is so strong that many physicians in a capitated system may not provide all the services they should, may not always be the patient's advocate, and may be reluctant to challenge the rules governing which services are appropriate. In fact, the health plan's contracts may forbid the doctors to disclose the existence of services not covered by the plan. This can pose "excruciating quandaries" (Beck 1995) for physicians. Soon many of them will find themselves conforming to the restrictions and deceiving themselves that what they are doing is best for their patients. So who stands for the customer (patient)? How about the quality of care? At that point, the true colors of managed care will be exposed.

To be competitive under managed care, one must continuously reduce expensive and unnecessary care as well as offer fewer services and reduce other types of waste. How do you do it? In the following chapters, the reader should find some of the answers that healthcare as a system needs to implement for true reform.

REFERENCES

JCAHO. *1995 Comprehensive Accreditation Manual for Hospitals.* Oakbrook Terrace, Ill.: Joint Commission on Accreditation of Healthcare Organizations, 1994.

Beck, J. "Managed Care May Jeopardize Your Health." *Detroit Free Press,* July 11, 1995, p. 9A.

Bryja, D. A.; R. D. Johannes; A. J. Kolod; J. R. Leach; R. Lee; D. P. Thornton; and M. S. Ulnick. "Strategies of a Global Company for Managing Fringe Benefit/Healthcare Costs into the 21st Century." In *Strategic Planning 2002: A Long-Run View.* Lansing, Mich.: Michigan State University Graduate School of Management, 1992.

PART ONE

Concepts, Theory, and Concerns of Quality in Healthcare

CHAPTER 1

Concerns of Quality in Healthcare

This chapter provides the reader with the foundation of what is really going on in healthcare. Specifically, it will address the issues of change, system thinking, strategic planning, and quality as they relate to healthcare. Furthermore, this chapter will define the concepts of process, customer, and variation from both a service and healthcare perspective.

PARADIGM CHANGE

We have long been taught that "the doctor knows best" and that "health facilities always provide you with the best care." In the 1990s and beyond, we are not so sure anymore. Sure, we believe the doctor and we trust the facility, but, at the same time, we also challenge them. The challenge may be in the diagnosis, test, hospital stay, and so on. Is this challenge because we have lost faith in the health system? Certainly not. We like to believe that we as customers (patients) can be active participants in our health. By the same token, the healthcare providers are concerned about productivity, costs, and profits. Our paradigms have indeed changed, and we are in the midst of drastic change.

In today's international business environment, increased productivity is a key to the economic success of nations, industries (both manufacturing and service), companies, and workers. Productivity can be determined by technology, work methods, choice of equipment, employees, and management. It is desirable to relate productivity to job satisfaction. Job satisfaction is based on the premise that workers need a quality or positive work experience to function properly. A decrease in job satisfaction can be translated into decreased productivity. Productivity is a measure of how well resources are combined and utilized to accomplish desirable results. In other words, productivity is the ratio of some output to some input. The essence, of course, is to do more with less. Output per work hour and bed utilization are some of the most common ways we measure productivity in healthcare. This output is influenced by many factors, which include the quality and availability of materials, the scale of operations and the rate of capacity utilization, the availability and put-through capacity of capital equipment, the attitude and skill level of the workforce, and the motivation and effectiveness of the management.

There are many theories regarding the productivity crisis in healthcare. Here, however, we are going to be concerned with the management and quality portions. One way to approach the productivity problem is through Abraham Maslow's (1943) needs hierarchy. According to Maslow, as lower needs are met, they become less important and less powerful motivators and higher level needs become activated. Maslow's contribution to solving the productivity problem is that his theory recognizes the importance of human needs in the work setting. This may be seen in Table 1–1.

TABLE   1–1

Application of Maslow's Hierarchy of Needs

Examples	Maslow's Hierarchy	Organizational Examples
Achievement	Self-actualization needs	Challenging job
Status	Esteem needs	Job title
Friendship	Belongingness	Friends in work group
Stability	Security needs	Pension plan
Sustenance	Physiological needs	Base salary

Frederick Herzberg (1959, 1968) proposed another theory to increase productivity and quality by making jobs more meaningful and giving the worker a voice in the design of his or her job. Herzberg's contribution to solving the productivity problem is that job factors can and may serve as a motivating function by providing job satisfaction. Herzberg talks about motivating factors as being intrinsic to the job, which include achievement, recognition for achievement, the work itself, responsibility, growth, and advancement. Also, factors extrinsic to the job are considered hygiene and include company policy and administration, supervision, interpersonal relationships, working conditions, salary, status, and security. Herzberg's conclusion was that extrinsic hygiene factors are primarily related to job satisfaction. This conclusion implies that management must maintain these hygiene factors, which promote professional growth, since management is responsible for these factors.

The implication so far leads us to believe that increases of productivity are a function of improved quality of work life (QWL). QWL is the extent to which employees are able to satisfy important needs through their work experience, with particular emphasis on participation in important decisions about their work. It is imperative, then, to break all the barriers within the organization, so that the work climate becomes hospitable to innovation. Organizations must adopt participatory management, eliminate bureaucratic layers of supervisors, listen to employees, and develop job security and retraining programs. Workers generally want to do a good job and will suggest work efficiencies if they feel that their job is secure.

Until recently, service quality has not been given as much priority as other considerations. For example, cost reduction, delivery, and overall production have taken precedence over quality and reliability. To understand this, we must examine the Alfred Sloan dictum. Sloan's thesis was laid down in the early 1920s and proclaimed that to gain market share against a competitor it is not necessary to have greater than competitive quality. The result is that management tolerated significant amounts of scrap, defective products, and the rework of defective products, along with an army of quality inspectors, checkers, rework, and repair personnel. This philosophy is symbolized by the acronym AQL, which stands

ble quality level. This philosophy stands in marked con-
_nat of modern quality thinking, which focuses on contin-
_nall-scale improvement, with the goal being elimination of
defe_ts. This continual improvement attitude has been refined by
Imai (1986) in his now famous Kaizen approach to productivity
success.

Another important contribution of modern quality thinking is
the notion of reengineering, which was introduced by Hammer
and Champy (1993) and emphasizes drastic changes. What is very
important, though, is that both Kaizen and reengineering teach
us that a quality superiority can be converted into higher price
and/or market share. The road to this achievement is through
three major areas: design engineering, supplier relations, and dif-
fusion of quality responsibility. Central to the strategy for each of
those major areas is a strong effort to get all employees to take responsibility for improved quality. Second, the strategy recognizes
that quality and productivity are not contrary objectives but mutually supportive ones. Third, it recognizes that quality is a carrier
for other desirable corporate objectives, such as employee involvement in decision making, inventory control, increased market
share, and, of course, productivity.

American companies, including those in healthcare, act as if
they have shaped their management cultures around the belief
that people are motivated primarily by money (Kovich 1993). Organizations believe that excellence of performance is stimulated by
competition among individuals. American organizations believe—
or seem to believe by their actions—that among all stakeholders,
the interests of stockholders predominate.

As grim as this makes American managers seem, it is a fact
that finally they have realized there is payback to giving workers
a say-so in what's going on in the company and the day-to-day operations. We see for the first time, even in service organizations,
that managers—

- Train their employees intensively, investing considerable
  sums in this, so that their value to the firm and to
  themselves never stagnates.
- Let the employees run their own workplace with
  considerable autonomy when they are operation workers;

they also let them make decisions affecting work procedure and improvements.

- Encourage the employees to attack problems and implement solutions through structures such as the quality control circles or the modern self-directed work teams (SDWTs) and through problem-solving techniques.
- Show trust in even larger ways; there is rotation of management and nonmanagement alike to gain knowledge and experience.
- Try to keep the workplace from being boring and depressing.

In healthcare, we are finally recognizing that quality involves the entire healthcare process—from the care given by the primary care physician, to the patient's laboratory, X-ray, and hospital experiences, to home care. However, the position of facilitator for the improvement in healthcare quality, no matter how defined, is a management responsibility and a function of leadership.

There is a lot of pressure for instant solutions, and U.S. healthcare management may not have the patience to continue with efforts that do not yield immediate results. Nevertheless, the pressures for U.S. healthcare providers to upgrade quality are intense, and some significant movement in that direction is apparent. Some of the movement is in the following areas:

1. Quality assurance personnel are receiving greater authority and are reporting to higher levels in the organization; this gives an added prominence and clout to the quality assurance effort.
2. At many facilities across the country, union and management representatives are sitting down and discussing the possibilities for cooperative activity in upgrading quality; in some cases, the cooperative effort has materialized in successful contractual agreements.
3. Greater attention is being paid to the quality of suppliers' goods.
4. Efforts are being made to improve coordination between cross-functional departments through advanced methods in statistical analysis.

5. Perhaps the most visible change is the extensive experimentation in training in areas such as statistical process control (SPC), problem solving, teams and SDWTs, design of experiments (DOE), benchmarking, quality function deployment (QFD), the Taguchi approach, cost of quality, failure mode and effect analysis (FMEA), control plans, and just-in-time inventory.

SYSTEM APPROACH

It seems that everyone involved with quality keeps talking about systems. However, no one, to my knowledge, has taken the time to address the issue from a quality perspective and especially from the healthcare perspective. So, let us start with the definition of system.

system

An arrangement of separate and independent components sharing a relationship for the purpose of attaining a common goal and predetermined objectives.

The system concept is a set of attitudes and a frame of mind rather than a definite and explicit theory. Application of the concept involves the use of logic, intelligence, and creativity. The system concept is increasingly becoming an important tool for reaching solutions to quality problems. Its major advantages are that it minimizes random trial and error methods, which can waste time, money, and other resources. It *forces* the recognition of the whole as being distinct from the subsystem elements. It insists that the problem be reviewed in its entirety by taking into account all facts (variables, constants, etc.) and relating them to the whole and each other (Novosad 1982).

System theory application is still considered an art. However, the mix of human intuition, mathematical precision, computer technology, and human experience has brought the system concept to a high plateau of rationality. All systems have the following common procedural aspects:

- The system concept demands the prior accounting of uncertainty in all strategic decisions.
- The system approach is reproducible.

- The system thinking approach to problem resolution recognizes the situation of avoidance; that is, when it is appropriate to avoid a particular issue because of extreme complexity or simplicity.
- Most system thinking approaches are used to generate appropriate and applicable questions.

Perhaps the most important attribute of the system concept is that it can be used by individuals and teams. Its strength is that it can radically challenge the status quo, regardless of its longevity in the work environment. In the quality field and more so in healthcare, problem solving must be accomplished in a systematic manner. We can no longer afford "the first way that works" or "that is the way we've always done it" solutions to our problem. *The Path of the Calf*, a poem, appears to be applicable in this regard.

> One day through the primeval wood
> A calf walked home as good calves should;
> But made a trail all bent askew,
> A crooked trail as all calves do.
> Since then 300 years have fled,
> And I infer the calf is dead.
> But still he left behind this trail
> And thereby hangs my moral tale.
> But the trail was taken up next day
> By a lone dog that passed that way;
> And then a wise bell-wether sheep
> Pursued the trail o'er vale and steep,
> And drew the flock behind him too,
> As good bell-wethers always do.
> And from that day, o'er hill and glade,
> Through those old woods a path was made,
> and many men would in and out
> And dodged and turned and bent about,
> And uttered words of righteous wrath
> Because 'was such a crooked path,
> But still they followed—do not laugh—
> The first migrations of that calf,
> And through this winding roadway stalked
> Because he wobbled when he walked.
> This forest path became a lane

That bent and turned and turned again;
This crooked lane became a road
Where many a poor horse with his load
Toiled beneath the burning sun,
And traveled some three miles in one;
And thus a century and a half
They trod in the footsteps of that calf.
The years passed on in swiftness fleet,
The road became a village street;
And this, before men were aware,
A city's crowded thoroughfare.
And soon the central street was this
Of a renowned metropolis;
And men two centuries and a half
Trod in the footsteps of that calf.
Each day a hundred thousand rout
Followed this zig-zag calf about;
And o'er his crooked journey went
The traffic of a continent.
A hundred thousand men were led
By one calf near three centuries dead.
They followed still his crooked way,
And lost one hundred years a day;
For thus such a reverence is lent
To well established precedent,
A moral lesson this might teach,
Were I ordained and called to preach.
For men are prone to go it blind
Along the calf paths of the mind,
And work away from sun to sun,
To do what other men have done.
They follow in the beaten track
And out and in, and forth and back,
And still their devious course pursue,
To keep the path that others do.
They keep the path and sacred groove
Along which all their lives they move,
But how the wise old wood-gods laugh
Who saw the first primeval calf.
Ah! Many things this tale might teach
But I am not ordained to preach.

Author Unknown

Characteristics of a System

A system can involve people, information, or things. At its simplest, a system can be described as a rational and orderly combination or arrangement of objectives, facts, or elements. Two of the most fundamental characteristics of the system are:

1. *Synergy.* Synergy is the term used to identify the behavior of whole systems unpredicted by the behavior of their parts taken separately. The catalyst for this synergy is coordination. In the formation of teams and SDWTs, we expect synergy through the coordination of effort on the part of the participants.

2. *System approach.* System approach is a holistic way of thinking that attempts to study the total or synergistic performance of a system before concentrating on the individual parts. This mode of operation recognizes that even if each element or subsystem is optimized individually from a design or functional viewpoint, the total system performance may be suboptimal owing to the interaction between the parts. Examples of using the system method in healthcare are everywhere. Two specific examples are in the implementation process of total quality management (TQM) and the training of management and nonmanagement personnel.

Knowledge of a System in Healthcare

Guiding an organization effectively toward continual improvement depends on the organization leaders' developing, basing their leadership on, and communicating to everyone the knowledge of the organization as a system of production, that is, a group of interdependent people, items, processes, and products and services that have a common purpose or aim (Batalden and Stoltz 1993; Bradford and Bradford 1993). To understand the work of the organization as a system of production and to manage for improvement, leaders must be able to answer and help others to answer three basic questions (Batalden and Stoltz 1993). They are:

Why we make what we make?
How we make what we make?
How we improve what we make?

Why we make what we make refers to the aim of the system. To answer this question requires developing and deepening customer knowledge as well as understanding the social need of the organization.

How we make what we make refers to the means of production. Answering this question requires building knowledge of what is actually created, made, or produced (services and products); how services or products are produced (processes); for whom they are produced (beneficiaries or customers); and on whom they depend (suppliers). In healthcare, as in other service industries, workers are accustomed to describing what they do everyday or the effects of their actions, not what they make.

How we improve what we make means developing knowledge of what must be done to improve toward a shared vision for the future (plan to improve) and formulating specific plans (design or redesign) based on these improvement priorities. Changes that will improve the overall system are those that increase the system's capacity to deliver services and products that meet the needs and expectations of the customers it seeks to serve.

For the purpose of continual improvement, understanding the interrelationship of the essential elements in the system is critical. Therefore, making wise decisions about what and how to improve requires linking knowledge of the various elements in a system (Ackoff 1984; Bertalanffy 1968; Checkland 1981; Mitroff 1988; Revans 1964; Senge 1990; Deming 1986). For example, key processes in a hospital are those required to produce information, diagnostic and therapeutic services, and the care environment. On the other hand, processes such as those relating to transportation, diet, and medical records contribute to the key processes at various points and may be referred to as supportive processes.

STRATEGIC PLANNING

Strategic planning is a systematic analysis of business situations evaluating both internal and external factors, as they will affect the current and future development of the organization. The analysis for the internal factors is focused on at least three issues. They are:

1. *Structure and nature of business activity.* Is the structure in

tune with the planning? Can the current structure support the proposed change? Is the structure compatible with the business?

2. *Available resources.* Does the organization have the resources to undergo the proposed change? If we do have the resources available, are we willing to allocate them for the suggested project? Can we afford the change now? What are the ramifications if we do not follow the change?

3. *Key capabilities and limitation.* Do we have the capability for change? Is our cultural attitude ready? Do we have the appropriate funding, support, and commitment from all concerned? Is our organization capable of the change?

On the other hand, the external factors are based on the following factors:

1. *Market segments.* Do we focus on a particular market, or do we try to be everything to everybody? Do our customers know that? Do they know the difference between our services and those of our competition?

2. *Competition.* Is our market saturated with similar services? How can we separate our services from those of our competition?

3. *Other factors beyond direct control.* Is our organization equipped with technological capabilities that the next closest facility offers? Is our supplier market competitive and available for optimizing costs? Are government regulations an inhibitor in our market? What are the general economic conditions of the surroundings? Is our location a factor?

Effective strategic planning must have a clear definition of what the business "should" be. To develop that clear definition, the organization must develop a vision, mission, specific strategies, a prioritization of goals and objectives, and an action plan. In addition, during the strategic implementation process, the appropriate time and resources should be allocated. To make sure that the strategic planning is working and is on target, a well-designed evaluation system must be in place to monitor the progress and development of the goals as set forth in the strategic plan. Figure 1–1 shows a typical matrix of selecting business strategies. Figure 1–2 shows a typical process of strategic planning, and Figure 1–3 shows the components for successful strategic planning.

A mission statement defines the intended future role of the business in terms of corporate commitment, strategic focus, mar-

FIGURE 1–1

General Business Strategies

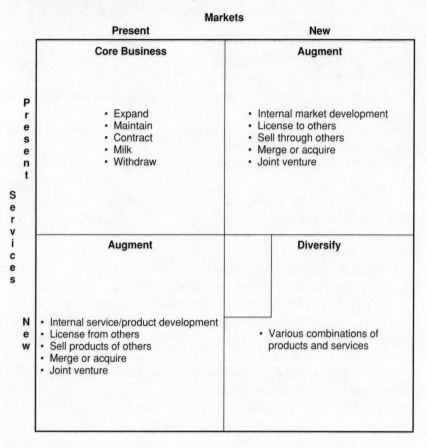

FIGURE 1–2

The Process of Strategic Planning

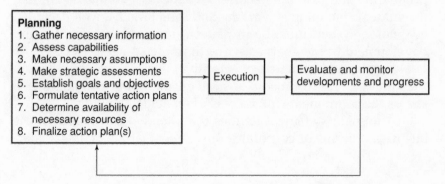

F I G U R E   1–3

Components for Successful Strategic Planning

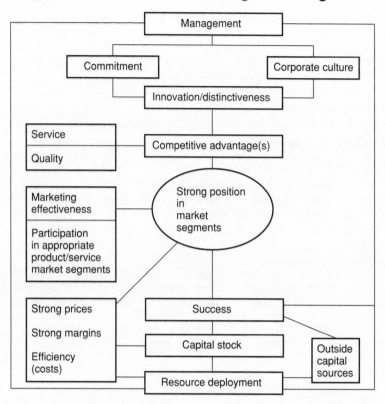

ket needs to be served, services or products to be provided, markets to be served, key competencies, and market identity. It must be remembered that any mission statement is an individualized statement and must be feasible (doable), desirable, and flexible. See Table 1–2 for an example of a mission statement.

Goals are general and continuing statements of intended future results. They are necessary and sufficient for the completion of individual tasks, and they can measure success. Objectives, on the other hand, are specific, measurable, time-related statements of intended future results. The accomplishment of objectives will lead to the attainment of the strategies, mission statement, and goals. All objectives must be important, challenging, and achievable. They should identify the priority, objective number and action plan leader. See Table 1–2 for examples of objectives and goals.

TABLE 1–2

Examples of Goals, Objectives, and a Mission Statement

Examples of Goals:

- Have a motivated, productive, and educated workforce with a high level of personal growth, pride, and satisfaction.
- Recognize and develop programs for customer satisfaction.
- Be competitive in the marketplace.
- Be the dominant force in the radiology field in our market.

Examples of Objectives:

- Develop a cost control system by 5/31/95.
- Develop a meaningful motivation program by 7/15/96.
- Develop appropriate acquisition procedures for machine purchases in the Radiology and Laboratory departments.
- Achieve job control of material usage in the Housekeeping and Maintenance Department.

Example of a Mission:

Thisvi Community Hospital (TCH) is an integral member of the Thisvi Community. It is our mission to provide quality healthcare to residents of our community. Beyond our mandated service area, we will always provide first-rate care to anyone in need of medical attention, regardless of race, religion, nationality, or ability to pay. As such, we provide a wide range of services:

- 24-hour emergency care
- A wide range of primary care outpatient services
- State-of-the art inpatient medical care, within a caring and patient-oriented environment

Through our role as a teaching hospital, TCH is dedicated to the development and dissemination of medical knowledge to patients and health professionals. TCH will provide the best public healthcare and, whenever appropriate, social services to the community that it serves.

Action plans are what translate wishes into results. An action plan should be written for each objective. Examples of different kinds of action plans are shown in Figures 1–4, 1–5, and 1–6. Typical action examples are as follows:

- Begin by filling in the heading for the action plan worksheet.
- List all the things that must be done to accomplish the objective.
- Rewrite the list of actions in proper time sequence.

F I G U R E   1–4

Blank Action Plan Form

Action Plan		
Objective:		
Activity	Required Resources	Time Schedule

- Number each action.
- Give each action a priority indicating the importance of the action.
- Indicate the status of each action.
- Identify the person(s) responsible for each action.
- Identify the preliminary cost for each action.

FIGURE 1–5

Typical Action Plan Form

Objective: **Priority:**
Objective #:   **Team Leader:**

Item number	Action	Priority	Dollars	Time	Team Involved	Start Date	Completion Date
1-1	Review training needs	1-U	$5,000	15	The Hawks		

Priority: 1–3, Critical; 4–6, Important; 7–9, Beneficial
Status: C = Complete; U = Underway; A = Approved; P = Proposed; T = Tentative

- Identify the preliminary time required for each person and for each action.
- Do not fill in the starting and completion dates until the action plan is scheduled in the final session.

F I G U R E   1–6

Sample Action Plan Form

Objective:	Priority Sequence	Responsibility	Action Plan Date—This Schedule _____ Date—Previous Schedule _____
Activity			Time Schedule

Warning! Action plans are team efforts and should never be initiated or completed by one individual. The action plan should not be a plan to plan but rather the specific action to achieve the objective. Action must be just that—action. An action statement should never be an intended outcome. It is a good practice for an action statement to begin with an action verb.

The purpose of strategic planning in the healthcare industry is based on the following principle: to sharply focus your organization's limited time and resources on the things that will truly maximize future profitability, survivability, and growth ability, without affecting patient care. As a consequence of this focus, the results expected are:

- A revelation of hidden pitfalls and risks.
- Help in dealing with future uncertainty.
- Help in becoming more opportunity oriented.
- Common understanding and coordination of effort.
- A means to reach agreement.
- Motivation, enthusiasm, and commitment built through involved participation.
- A boost in morale because the participants belong to an organization that knows where it is going.
- Relief of anxieties by making known the previously unknown and dealing with any problems or challenges.
- Help in reaching higher levels of attainment.
- A coordinated business plan, which lenders and investors will find attractive.
- A stronger competitive position.

Some useful competitive strategies in healthcare are shown in Table 1–3. Figures 1–7 and 1–8 show, respectively, how specialty versus commodity indicators and positioning in healthcare are defined and how one may go about defining a competitive strategy. The question that the reader may have by now is, If strategic planning is so great, why is it that some healthcare institutions have faulty plans—attributed to not having enough time—or they do not plan at all? The reason may be any one or a combination of the following:

- Some people consider strategic planning as a manufacturing tool that does not apply to healthcare.
- Some feel that it is superfluous because they know clearly where they are going.

T A B L E   1–3

Useful Competitive Strategies for Healthcare

Clear differentiation
Gain a strong market share within a market segment
Avoid head-to-head confrontation wherever possible
Customize services
Market a problem solver image
Respond quickly to important changes in the marketplace
Be responsive to your organization's corporate culture
Focus on long-term growth, rather than short-term profit
Focus on high value-added services
Define a market niche and go after it
Avoid financial overextension
Market specific services and the services embodied in your organization's
  capabilities, technology, resources, and vision

- Strategic planning is sometimes viewed as something for big business only.
- Some leaders seem to prefer one-man, seat-of-the-pants planning.
- There is sometimes a concern that strategic planning will be time consuming.
- There may be a fear of failure due to lack of knowledge and skills.
- Some believe that uncertainty renders planning useless.
- Some organizations just never getting around to making a strategic plan.

To be sure, there are potential pitfalls in strategic planning. As most of them are self-explanatory, they are offered without commentary:

- Failure to get started.
- Adoption of a complex planning model.
- Failure to establish and adhere to a schedule.
- Selection of an inappropriate leader or one with a personal agenda.

F I G U R E   1–7

Specialty versus Commodity Indicators and Positioning in Healthcare

	Specialty	Commodity
Indicators	• Unique service • Superiority due to superb marketing • Sales due to having the "right" service • Strong margins/profits	• Little differentiation • Substitutability • Sales due to low price • Sales due to location • Weak margins
Positioning	• Value-based pricing • Exceed customer requirements • High level of customer support	• Competitive pricing • Meet customer requirements

- Exclusive concentration on threats and weaknesses.
- Mechanical application of planning theory.
- Allowing planning to become mere budgeting and forecasting.
- Failure to integrate strategic planning into regular management process.
- Failure to monitor developments and process.
- Failure to prepare the CEO for his or her proper role in the process.
- Planning without the CEO's active participation.
- Doing your homework at the last minute.

FIGURE   1–8

Competitive Strategy

	Broad Overall Markets	Marketing Niches (selected narrow segments)
	Differentiation	**Segmentation**
Specialty Status (services that command premiums)	• Uniqueness • Service recognition • High marketing **High volume/High margins**	• Special features service • Emphasis on customization • High visibility of price **Low volume/High margins**
	Low Cost/Price	**Price**
Commodity Status (routine services that command low price)	• Economies of scale • Standardization • No frills • High visibility of price **High volume/Low margins**	• Cheapness • Strictly price orientation **Low volume/Low margins**

- Allowing strategic planning to become operational planning.
- Sole dependence on an untested supplier.
- Promoting achievement beyond level of competence.
- Acceptance of downside risks that should not be accepted.
- Believing everything the customer/supplier/competitor tells you.

So, how do we go about planning for an effective strategic plan? We follow two steps. First, we identify the factors that lead to the initiation of planning. From a generic perspective they are:

- New opportunities.
- New threats.

- Change in management team.
- Rapid growth.
- Stagnation.
- New problems.
- Uncertainty.
- Disagreement among principals.
- Need for major funding.
- Need for team building.
- General dissatisfaction of employees and management.

Second, we identify the specific focus within our organization that will help us develop a successful strategic plan. Correct strategic focus is the most important single element in success because it multiplies the effectiveness of limited time and resources. From a generic perspective the plan should follow these guidelines:

A. Sound approach
   1. Logical framework
   2. Planning schedule
   3. Simplicity
B. Commitment and involvement of top management
C. Integration into "own" management process
D. Enthusiasm
E. Good planning leadership
   1. Understanding of planning process
   2. Conceptual ability
   3. Objectivity
   4. Leadership skills
   5. Communication skills
   6. Broad perspective
F. Time and money
E. Evaluation

Are we better or worse off, or are we the same?

DEFINITION OF QUALITY

The word *quality* when used to describe products or services creates many images in the minds of different people. It could be the image of a Cadillac, Rolls Royce, Saks Fifth Avenue, Lenox china,

a grade A prime steak, the Cleveland Clinic, a.
ity products or services are perceived to be bett.
more reliable, and usually more costly than those ι.
Crosby (1979) has declared that quality is free and it .
quality that really has large costs associated with it.

The American service industry is now beginning to se   .e
of the importance of quality. This importance is apparent iι. the
healthcare industry in which, for many years, everything was all
right as long as cost plus profit was the modus operandi. Lately,
however, that premise has been challenged, and healthcare is looking for answers in effectiveness of service and profitability, in the
world of quality. So what is quality all about? Webster's dictionary
defines it as:

---
quality

Any of the features that make something what it is; characteristics; attributes
Basic nature; character; kind
The degree of excellence a thing possesses
Excellence; superiority

There are many other definitions of quality. For example, some define it as a measure of how closely a good or service conforms to
specified standards (Tersine 1985). Others define it as a conformance to requirements (Crosby 1979). Others define it as the degree to which a specified product or service satisfies the wants of
a specific consumer. Yet others define it as the degree to which a
specific product or service is preferred over competing products of
equivalent grade, based on comparative tests by consumers (Juran
1962). Continual improvement is another definition of quality
(Deming 1986). Quality as defined by the customer is another
(Ford 1990). Loss to society is a further definition (Taguchi 1987).

What emerges from all these definitions of quality and what
is important is that the term *quality* is elusive and difficult to define
in specific terms. The general attitude "I'll know it when I see it"
somehow has a true ring to it. The fact is, quality is much more
than the preceding definitions can describe or will allow the reader
to interpolate. In the final analysis, especially in healthcare, we believe that quality is an issue of personal perception but that it is
also an issue of value. For an extensive discussion on this issue, see
Stamatis (1995a) and Garvin (1988). Here I will briefly explain perception versus value.

The real or perceived excellence of the product or service may make it appealing to a customer. It may also result in the willingness of the customer to pay premium prices for the product or service, as this aspect of quality is considered to increase. The value of quality is composed of the parts, the value in the design, and the value in the conformance to that design (Juran 1962). The value associated with design is referred to by Juran as *grade*. Grade may be related to such factors as appearance, extent of required maintenance, reliability, interchangeability, luxury of features, and safety factors. The cost of value can be many times recovered through the price of the product or service while occasionally even increasing demand. Grade may be actively sought after and may create a willingness in the customer to pay premium prices in the belief that value is determined through the factors that determine grade rather than the basic operation of the product or service. This may result in the purchase of a more costly product or service than one that would function equally well but has not established itself as a quality item. However, as a result of improper or inadequate market survey or creation of requirements, the added value does not always provide an increased worth to the consumer. If this is true, the cost will not be recovered and may become a detrimental cost of quality instead.

The goal of quality is to achieve superior external and internal customer satisfaction levels. However, regardless of how one defines quality, one thing is certain. The fundamental precepts of quality are always the same for any industry and always remain flexible, so that they can change with the expectations of the customer. To summarize, the precepts of quality are as follows:

- Quality excellence can best be achieved by preventing problems, rather than by detecting and correcting them after they occur.
- All work that is done by employees, suppliers, and providers is part of a process that creates a product or service for a customer. Each person can influence some part of that process and, therefore, affect the quality of its output and ultimately the customers' satisfaction with products and services.
- Sustained quality excellence requires continuous improvement. This means, regardless of how good present performance may be, it can become even better.

- Each employee is a customer for work done by other employees or suppliers or providers, with a right to expect good work from others and an obligation to contribute work of high caliber to those who, in turn, are his or her customers.
- Quality is—more often than not—defined by the customer; the customer wants products and services that, throughout life, meet his or her needs and expectations at a cost that represents value.
- People provide the intelligence and generate the actions that are necessary to realize all improvements.

Finally, we must always remember that the issue of quality and the patient is a sensitive one and how we define that relationship is only circumstantial. In real terms, regardless of what definition we give to quality, regardless of what the Joint Commission on Accreditation of Healthcare Organizations demands of our healthcare delivery, regardless of what the governmental regulations state, regardless of what a third-party certification says about the quality system, regardless of what quality system we have or what we think of our own quality system, the patient perceives quality in the context of his or her own experience.

THE CONCEPT OF PROCESS

Traditionally, a process has been defined as follows:

process

A series of actions that repeatedly come together to transform inputs provided by a supplier into outputs received by a customer

Output is simply what is produced by the actions. Actions that repeatedly come together are a combination of all or part of the following:

- Manpower (people)
- Machines (technology)
- Method
- Material
- Measurement
- Environment

The focus of this process is to generate an output given an input. The greater the ratio of that output to input, the more efficient the operation is. This can be seen in Figure 1–9. This figure represents a generic process model, which visually represents the process in relationship to its components.

In healthcare three additional attributes are associated with the term *process*. They are:

- *Structure*—The sources put together to deliver the service.
- *Process*—The service itself.
- *Outcomes*—The value results of the service.

The focus of this process is to generate the outcome (benefit), which meets or exceeds the needs, wants, and expectations of the customer. Figure 1–10 shows the relationship of a traditional service process and its components as well as the appropriate fit of the customer. Figure 1–11 shows a typical process example from a healthcare environment, using the Deming philosophy. (For the basic philosophy of Deming, see Appendix A.) What is interesting about the service process definition is that within the structure, process, and outcomes, we may indeed have to account for the traditional components of the manufacturing process.

Another important quality issue in healthcare is the concern of the owner. Who is the real owner of the process? The owner turns out to be the same as in the traditional manufacturing environment. That is, the owner of the process is the person who has or is given the responsibility and authority to lead the continuing improvement of a given process. Process ownership is driven by the boundaries of the process. For example:

Individual process ←————————→ Individual ownership

A task performer is the responsible party for accountability and responsibility for that individual task.

Functional process ←————————→ Unit-based ownership

A bundle of individual processes is the responsibility of the department supervisor, who has both the responsibility and accountability for the entire department.

Cross-functional processes ←————————→ Unclear ownership

Although theoretically the responsibility and accountability are present, even in this highly structured environment, in reality, as you move away from the individual process, that authority and responsibility are diffused throughout the processes.

FIGURE 1-9

Generic Process Model

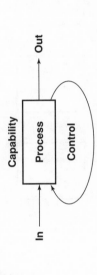

Capability

In → **Process** → Out

Control

Where the IN are:
• Manpower
• Machines
• Methods
• Material
• Measurement
• Environment

Where the PROCESS is:
• The transformation of the IN to the reason of existence (e.g., glass making, hotel service, insurance service)

Where the CONTROL is:
• The mechanism for ensuring that the process is producing what is expected

Where CAPABILITY is:
• The ability of the process to perform up to the expected performance

Where the OUT is:
• The finished service

FIGURE   1–10

Traditional Method of Ensuring Service Quality

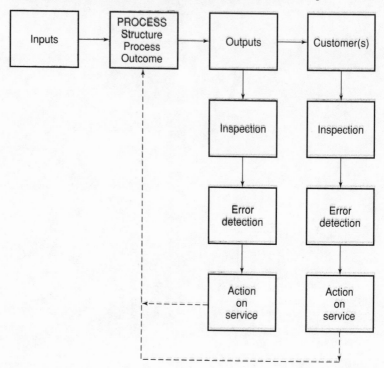

Another unique characteristic about the healthcare process is the fact that quite often processes operate both sequentially and in parallel at the same time. Thus, of course, it is more difficult and becomes more complicated to precisely define the boundaries of "the" process. An example of this is a patient entering the hospital through the emergency department. While the patient is in the emergency room, other departments, such as the Intensive Care Unit (ICU), are also required to be present or involved with the delivered care (Figure 1–12). Figure 1–13 demonstrates the complexity and various components of a system of production in healthcare.

Process Control

The effort to control a process and its output consists of essentially four elements:

   1. *The process.* The combination of people, machines (technol-

FIGURE   1–11

Deming's Method of Service Quality—Extended Process

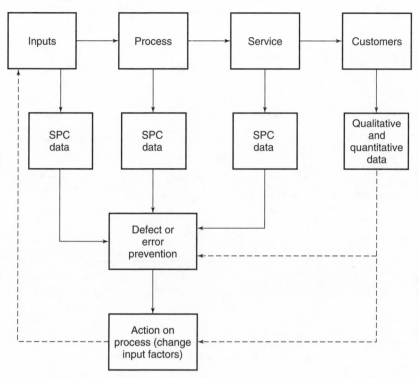

ogy), materials, methods, measurement, and work environment works together to produce output. The total performance of the process—the quality of its output and its productive efficiency—depends on the way the process has been designed and built, and on the way it is operated. The rest of the process control system is useful only if it contributes to improved performance of the process.

2. *Information about performance.* Much information about the actual performance of the process can be learned by studying the process output. In a broad sense, process output includes not only the products and services but also any intermediate "outputs" that describe the operating state of the process, such as cycle time and response time. If this information is gathered and interpreted correctly, it can show whether action is necessary to correct the process or the just-produced output. If timely and appropriate actions are not taken, however, any information-gathering effort is wasted.

FIGURE 1–12

Relationship of the Customer in Healthcare

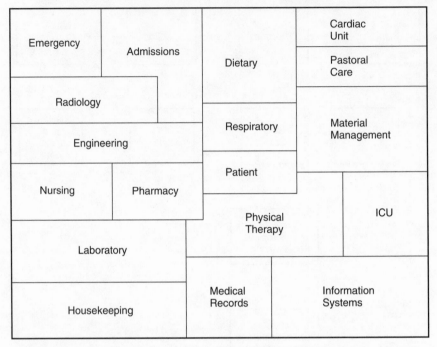

Note: There is no linearity. A given supplier may service more than one customer independent of all other departments, vertically and/or horizontally.

3. *Action on the process.* This area is future oriented and is taken when necessary to prevent the output from being out-of-specification. This action may consist of changes in the operations (training, method of doing the task, material, etc.) or the more basic elements of the process itself as a whole. The effect of actions should be monitored, and further analysis and action should be taken if necessary.

4. *Action on the output.* This area is past oriented because it involves detecting out-of-specification outputs already produced. Unfortunately, if current output does not consistently meet specification, it may be necessary to sort all products and to scrap or re-work any nonconforming items. This must continue until the necessary corrective action on the process has been taken and verified, or until the specification has been changed.

F I G U R E   1–13

**Typical Hospital View as a System Capable
of Continual Improvement**

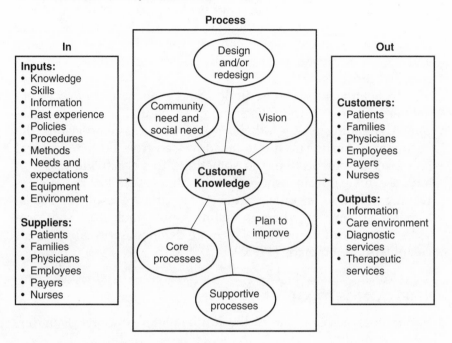

As is probably obvious, action on the process is the most crucial element in the area of process control. Unlike action on the
output, it involves preventing rather than producing and sorting
and second-guessing nonconforming units and nonconformities.
The major tool used in this effort is the process control chart (see
Chapter 5).

THE CONCEPT OF CUSTOMER

customer

Anyone inside or outside your work environment who receives your organization's
product or service

In healthcare, as in many other service organizations, there are
several categories of customers. These include patients, physicians, nurses, government, insurers, the community, employees,

and families and friends of the patients, among others. Each of these groups may evaluate the quality of care delivery using different criteria. For example, good delivery of care may be evaluated by the patient on the basis of bedside manners of the physician and the nurse. On the other hand, the physician may evaluate the care based on the latest technology used. The patient's family and friends may evaluate the care by the amount of time the physician and nurse spent with them.

In healthcare we must understand that the customer's care delivery process is multidisciplinary in nature, with each discipline depending on the others. Because of this relationship, the customer in healthcare has to be addressed from both an internal and external perspective, and sometimes this is difficult to do. In any case, in healthcare especially, a customer is not just the money-waving ultimate consumer (patient) of healthcare resources. A customer is anyone anywhere to whom you or your work unit provides service or information. For more detailed information about customers, see Stamatis (1995a).

THE CONCEPT OF VARIATION

Variation is perhaps one of the fundamental concepts of understanding quality.

variation

Difference between a measurement point and a target point

Everything—people, processes, and objects—has variation. To say that something has no variation is to say that something is perfect all the time every time.

In quality, when one speaks of variation, it is necessary to separate the two kinds of variation that exist. The first kind, random, inherent, or common variation, exists all the time in everything; the second kind, the assignable or special variation, exists because of a specific reason. Random variation, generally speaking, cannot be removed from the process unless the process is changed. On the other hand, special variation is the result of disruptions to the process, which usually can be removed by people working in the process.

Whereas in manufacturing variation is a straightforward experience, in healthcare, it sometimes presents difficulties. For example, in food preparation, quality may be affected by the temperature of the oven or the texture of the fruit, and yet it may not be feasible to establish tight tolerances on these characteristics. Similarly, it is usually not possible to control the quality (types) of patients entering your healthcare facility. Some patients may be hard of hearing; some will have special needs or be more demanding than others. The number of customers seeking service, as well as the medical treatment delivered, is also difficult to control. And if there is bad weather or an electrical power failure, it may be possible to close a manufacturing plant for the day, but not the healthcare facility. For these reasons, it is imperative to think of variation in healthcare as three distinct types:

1. *Assignable variation.* This type of variation is a disruption of the process, which can be removed and possibly be prevented.
2. *Intrinsic random variation.* This type of variation is a collection of many minor sources of variation which are part of the process.
3. *Extrinsic random variation.* This type of variation can be disruptions of the usual process or operation but are not preventable, removable, or controllable.

For a detailed discussion on variation, see Wheeler (1993); for a discussion on the human error contribution to variation, see Stamatis (1995b).

REFERENCES

Ackoff, R. L. *Creating the Corporate Future.* New York: John Wiley & Sons, 1984.
Batalden, P. B., and P. K. Stoltz. "A Framework for the Continual Improvement of Healthcare: Building and Applying Professional and Improvement Knowledge to Test Changes in Daily Work." *Journal on Quality Improvement,* October 1993, pp. 424–45.
Bertalanffy, L. *General Systems: Foundations, Development, Applications.* New York: Braziller, 1968.
Bradford, C. L., and R. W. Bradford. *Simplified Strategic Planning.* Vero Beach, Fla.: Center for Simplified Strategic Planning, 1993.
Checkland, P. *Systems Thinking, System Practice.* New York: John Wiley & Sons, 1981.

Crosby, P. B. *Quality Is Free*. New York: McGraw-Hill, 1979.

Deming, W. E. *Out of the Crisis*. Cambridge, Mass.: Massachusetts Institute of Technology, 1986.

Ford Motor Co. *Planning for Quality*. Dearborn, Mich.: Ford Motor Co., Corporate Quality Office, 1990.

Garvin, D. A. *Managing Quality*. New York: Free Press, 1988.

Hammer, M., and J. Champy. *Reengineering the Corporation*. New York: Harper Business, 1993.

Herzberg, F. "One More Time: How Do You Motivate Employees?" *Harvard Business Review*, January–February 1968, pp. 53–62.

Herzberg, F.; B. Mausner; and B. Snyderman. *The Motivation to Work*. New York: John Wiley & Sons, 1959.

Imai, M. *Kaizen: The Key to Japan's Competitive Success*. New York: Random House Business Division, 1986.

Juran, J. M. *Quality Control Handbook*. New York: McGraw-Hill, 1962.

Kovich, S. "What Employees Want." *Quality Digest*, March 1993, p. 32.

Maslow, A. H. "A Theory of Human Motivation." *Psychological Review* 50 (1943), pp. 374–96.

Mitroff, I. I. *Break-Away Thinking*. New York: John Wiley & Sons, 1988.

Novosad, J. P. *Systems, Modeling and Decision Making*. Dubuque, Ia.: Kendal/ Hunt Publishing, 1982.

Revans, R. W. *Standards for Morale: Cause and Effect in Hospitals*. London: Oxford University Press, 1964.

Senge, P. M. *The Fifth Discipline: The Art and Practice of the Learning Organization*. New York: Doubleday, 1990.

Stamatis, D. H. *Total Quality Service*. Delray Beach, Fla.: St. Lucie Press, 1995a.

———. *Failure Mode and Effect Analysis: FMEA from Theory to Execution*. Milwaukee: Quality Press, 1995b.

Taguchi, G. *System of Experimental Design*. Vols. 1–2. White Plains, N.Y.: UNIPUB/ Kraus International Publications, 1987.

Tersine, R. J. *Production/Operations Management: Structure and Analysis*. New York: Elsever Science Publishing, 1985.

Wheeler, D. J. *Understanding Variation: The Key to Managing Chaos*. Knoxville, Tenn.: SPC Press, 1993.

CHAPTER 2

Overview of Total Quality Management in Healthcare

This chapter gives an overview of the TQM philosophy and provides both a generic model and a healthcare model for TQM. The details of the implementation process will be discussed in Chapter 12.

FOLLOWING THE YELLOW BRICK ROAD

In the *Wizard of Oz*, when Dorothy realized that she was no longer in Kansas, she desperately wanted to return home. However, the Munchkins told her that she must go to Oz to see the great wizard. Only the wizard could return her to Kansas. To get to Oz, Dorothy would have to follow the yellow brick road. Along her trip to Oz, Dorothy encountered many problems and took them with her, so that the wizard would cure them.

In some respects many healthcare executives are just like Dorothy. They woke up from the profitable and comfortable early 1980s to find the 90s fraught with problems of increasing government intervention, customer demands for lower healthcare costs, rising costs of doing business, and lower reimbursements. Now healthcare executives are faced with "following the yellow brick road" to return home. They are looking for the help of a wizard to return them to a secure business status. Is that secure business status going to be accomplished by total quality management (TQM)?

Many healthcare executives believe that TQM is, in fact, the wizard. They are jumping on that "yellow brick road," and they are looking for fast, accurate, and real solutions on their journey. As it turns out, that road is the implementation process of TQM, and by the time we reach the wizard we will have implemented TQM in the organization.

THE TRANSITION INTO TQM

TQM has been one of the biggest changes to come to the healthcare community. Long a fundamental part of the business and manufacturing industries, TQM now is having a tremendous impact on the health industry as well. What is interesting about this adaptation is that many of the same reasons that drove the manufacturing industry to TQM are the same driving factors for healthcare. Healthcare is finding that it is being faced with decreasing profits, problems with employee relations, and problems with productivity. Furthermore, as an industry, healthcare has been portrayed in the media as "a bunch of hungry, greedy" professionals who will stop at nothing in the name of profit. The media, in fact, has pronounced the healthcare system itself as the villain. This has caused a decrease in patient satisfaction and an overall perception of poor quality. In addition, it has brought the wrath of politicians for a quick fix and reform.

To be sure, healthcare has become a costly fringe benefit for business and industry. According to Rooney (1989), the U.S. business world is spending 30 percent of its revenues on healthcare. Since 1989 this cost has been accelerating, which has forced many businesses to look for alternatives. The alternatives, however, have brought their own problems, including quality issues. To diffuse the situation, some businesses have begun to form partnerships with healthcare providers to reduce costs and to buy the care directly, rather than going through a third party (insurance). This partnering relationship has created a new concept in healthcare. All of a sudden we talk about "customers" and "suppliers," as opposed to strictly patients, doctors, nurses, facilities, and so on. The introduction of the "customer" and "supplier" concepts demands that certain standards be followed and the needs, wants, and expectations of the customer be identified and addressed.

This approach more or less "forced" healthcare into the world of TQM beginning in the late 1980s. This does not mean that before TQM was introduced, there was no quality or that the needs of the customer were not recognized. To the contrary, quality has always been an issue in healthcare, but it was of the mentality "doctors know best." It was a mentality that quality is only an issue of patient care. It focused on the diagnosis and intervention or treatment the patient received. It did not address the process of delivering patient care. With TQM, this old paradigm is changing and is focusing on team synergy to provide the best possible care to the patient.

Some reasons why the "forcing" took place are reports of poor quality practices in the following:

- Laboratory services (increased demand for specific tests but not enough technologists to perform the tests; incorrect diagnoses of Pap smears, tests for cancer, etc.).
- Pharmaceutical industries (controlling the drug market for profit, e.g., Prozac).
- Medical devices (introducing devices without thorough testing or without telling all the research results, e.g., breast implants).
- Hospital facilities (patients having the wrong surgeries, receiving wrong medications, etc.).

The notoriety of such incidents attracted the attention of the legislators, who in 1988 passed the Clinical Laboratory Improvement Act. As a direct result of this legislation, many changes have occurred, especially changes in quality. These changes, by necessity, have looked toward TQM for guidance and improvement.

Another reason why TQM is a viable alternative in healthcare is because of the patient. Patients have their own definition of what quality is. More often than not, the patient as a customer not only does not know what is happening but also is not even aware of good medical practice. The patient's only interest is to eliminate his or her pain and illness. Yet, as changes in attitude toward quality have emerged, so has the tolerance of what the customer will accept. Legislation has made it that much easier for litigation when the customer is dissatisfied with quality, however that quality is defined. Litigation has proved to be extremely costly for health-care; many healthcare facilities have closed down, and numerous physicians have been driven out of their practices. These lawsuits often have resulted in very high monetary settlements as well as increased internal costs for overcautiousness to prevent future litigation.

When healthcare executives began to look at TQM as the new corporate philosophy, many were merely jumping on a band-wagon. They were imitators of the next organization, and they viewed the concept of TQM as nothing more than a fad in management. After all, it sounds good to spout off the appropriate TQM jargon at a gathering of executive peers, proving that your company is indeed totally immersed in TQM principles. However, healthcare has become an extremely competitive industry, and TQM is now viewed as a survival issue for any organization for the 90s and beyond. Healthcare executives are looking at Deming's success in manufacturing and are realizing that their problems of improving service and productivity, decreasing overall costs, and increasing market share can be smoothed out by the introduction of TQM principles. For the first time, healthcare professionals are realizing that their problems follow a certain pattern and are not exclusively technical issues. TQM principles can and are being spread throughout all hospital areas—from housekeeping to nursing to radiology to the emergency department to medical floors and to physicians.

However, there appears to be a panic alarm sounding from the healthcare industry that TQM is the "911" response team being called on to rescue the industry. Healthcare has tried other programs, such as quality circles, the governance program, productivity studies and service excellence, and participative management with no significant results. So what is it about TQM that will make it work? To answer this question, we must look at the two major components of healthcare: (1) physicians and (2) the structure of the organization (process, outcome, etc.).

Physicians' active participation in total quality management is almost guaranteed by the fact that physicians, as providers of healthcare, receive approximately 20 percent of the total healthcare dollars, and the decisions they make generate the remaining 80 percent of that health dollar (Rooney 1992). Those decisions include hospitalization, laboratory tests, pharmaceuticals, and physical therapy. It seems only natural that physicians' contribution to the change process is important and must not be sidetracked. TQM will facilitate this participation without fear or intimidation to the healthcare system.

This second component of healthcare will also benefit from the implementation of TQM. TQM will provide the entire organization with specific improvement outcomes in areas such as quality of care, productivity, employee satisfaction, community perceptions, patient satisfaction, market share, net income, and physician satisfaction. Although these promised improvements may sound like utopia, Greene (1992), in his now famous Chicago health executive forum of 16 healthcare organizations, found that indeed these items can result from a TQM effort.

The next question, then, is, What are the ways to ensure success and survival? There are many steps that healthcare professionals can take to ensure that their TQM efforts are not in vain or that, once implemented, they will not be forgotten. Perhaps the first step is to assess the readiness and climate of the organization. You cannot suddenly say, "From now on we operate under TQM principles." The organization must be ready for such an introduction. If preparations are not appropriate, there is a guaranteed failure waiting to happen. Just as the farmer tills and fertilizes the ground before sowing it, so the leadership of the organization must identify where the organization is. This can be accomplished through a self-assessment, employee surveys, interviews, audits, and so on. Each method has its own advantages and disadvantages. Regardless of which method the organization uses, the intent is to learn more about the internal organization, management style, level of commitment, and receptiveness to accept change. The rationale for such knowledge is that if management knows in advance where the problems are or may occur, they may plan for appropriate resolution (Bell 1993).

The second essential part of transition into TQM involves communication and commitment. Management must openly communicate and daily demonstrate to *all* employees its commitment to TQM. Houghton (1992) describes this important part of TQM implementation as, "I have tried to make my feet match the walk." Houghton further explains that he tries to visit between 40 and 50 of his company's facilities every year speaking primarily on quality. Failure to communicate can cause employee morale to decline. When true commitment is not present, everyone is "doing their thing" without regard to synergy and improvement for the whole organization. The results of such behaviors may turn out to be poor service to the customer, which results in a perception of poor quality.

A third essential element of TQM implementation is the concern of education. By industry standards, healthcare uses some of the most educated and most specially trained employees. Why then, do employees need more education and training? Medical techniques, technology, tests, drugs, and treatments are changing all the time and, as a consequence, education and training are part of this ever continuing process. With TQM, it is no different; education and training are an ongoing pursuit. This education and training must be on a "just-in-time" basis so that the philosophy, tools, expectations, and fine-tuning become real instruments in the improvement process. One of the basic aspects of this education is the notion that the organization must begin to operate in a data-driven manner. In other words, management must begin to operate by facts. To do this, management is responsible for establishing measurable standards and expectations (objectives).

A fourth essential element of TQM implementation is the development of a strategic plan. Without a plan, the best of intentions could be fragmented, efforts duplicated, and both time and money wasted. Knowing where you want to go requires knowledge of what is going on inside and outside your organization. The gaining of inside knowledge is accomplished with surveys, audits, interviews, and the like. It is internally dependent. The "outside knowledge" is accomplished with benchmarking, quality function deployment, and so on. It is externally dependent. An important issue of strategic planning is the fact that, even though your organization may use it, there is no guarantee of success. What is guaranteed is that the organization must be prepared to continually develop the strategy that will lead to the ultimate destination. This preparation may take the form of modification or drastic change.

In essence, then, TQM offers a systematic method as well as a philosophy for a transformation of individuals and the organization as a whole. This transformation in its simplest form may be summarized as a change from traditional thinking to new TQM thinking (Table 2–1). It is a fresh approach for healthcare managers, and it is certainly a fresh approach for those being managed. The best news is that the principles of TQM can produce quality improvements for both the individual and the organization.

A GENERIC MODEL OF TQM

In organizations that implement the TQM philosophy, major changes will occur. Some of the obvious changes are in:

- The way we think.
- Our corporate culture.
- How we view and treat the customers.
- How we view and treat our employees.
- How we view and treat our community.
- How we view and treat shareholder relationships.

T A B L E   2–1

Traditional versus TQM Thinking

Traditional Thinking	TQM Thinking
Quality improvement is management's responsibility	Quality improvement is everyone's responsibility
Customers are outsiders we sell to	Customers (internal and external) are vital components of our organization
Good enough is good enough	Nothing less than 100% effort will do
We need better people to improve our quality	We already have the best people for the job
Vendors and suppliers are our adversaries	Vendors and suppliers are important members of our team
Quality comes from inspection, rejection, and rework	Quality is built into products and services from the start
"If it ain't broke, don't fix it"	"If it ain't broke, improve it." Continuous improvement is the *only* way
Quality improvement is expensive and labor intensive	Quality improvement reduces cost and increases productivity

But what is TQM? When we break down or examine each of the words, the message is loud and clear. *Total* implies at every level in the company, each and every day, in every department and support group. *Quality* indicates continuous improvement to meet and/or exceed internal or external customer requirements and expectations. *Management* occurs by establishing systems and environments that support a continuous improvement culture. Thus, the following definition applies.

total quality management

A strategic, integrated management system, which involves all managers and employees and uses quantitative methods to continuously improve an organization's processes to meet and exceed customer needs, wants, and expectations

There are five assumptions required to implement TQM:

1. *Customer focus.* The customers—both internal and external—must be identified and their needs must be understood. To do this, customer requirements must be established, and some kind of compliance must be in place. Finally, there must be a partnering relationship with key customers and suppliers, so that appropriate and applicable operationalization of the requirements will take place. At every step in the process, there is a customer and a supplier. A supplier is defined as the one who passes on the customer, patient, information, material, and so on. A customer is one who receives the customer, patient, information, material and so on. Depending on the task and the level of the organization, it is not unusual to see a customer treated as a supplier and a supplier treated as a customer. For more on this point, see Stamatis (1995).

2. *Total involvement* (commitment). Management must demonstrate the commitment and leadership through real opportunities for quality improvement for all employees, and it must appropriately delegate and empower employees to improve their work environment through creation of multidisciplinary, cross-functional, and self-directed teams.

3. *Measurement.* Management must establish a baseline measure with customers and develop the appropriate process and results measure. To develop this, the proper input and output criteria must be identified, so that a relationship of congruence is established between customer requirements and process variables.

If there is no congruence of the requirements and the process, correction and improvement are in order.

4. *Systematic support.* Management is responsible for managing the quality process. To do that, it must do two things. First, it must build a quality infrastructure tied to the internal management structure. Second, it must link quality to existing management systems, unless proven unworthy of continuing the upkeep of such systems.

5. *Continuous improvement.* Perhaps one of the most fundamental issues of TQM is that management must recognize and preach that *all* work must be viewed as a process. As such, it is management's responsibility to anticipate changes as well as the ramifications of the needs, wants, and expectations of customers, employees, and society. The changes should be in either a Kaizen (incremental) or reengineering (drastic) format, as found appropriate in the given organization. To be successful at this, the focus is on reduction of cycle time (in all processes) as well as encouraging and gladly receiving appropriate and timely feedback.

These responsibilities and assumptions are shown in the TQM model in Figure 2–1. The figure shows that the basis for TQM is indeed management through leadership. A TQM leader's function is to:

- Create a vision and establish a mission for the organization.
- Set realistic quality improvement goals.
- Identify the appropriate customers and their needs, wants, and expectations.
- Lead the culture change to a team environment.
- Serve on a strategic planning committee.
- Serve on the quality steering committee.
- Lead the improvement effort throughout the organization.
- Provide the opportunity to form teams.
- Recognize the need for both education and training.
- Train the employees.
- Empower the employees to resolve issues affecting their own work.
- Encourage the employees to participate without fear.

FIGURE 2–1

Generic TQM Model

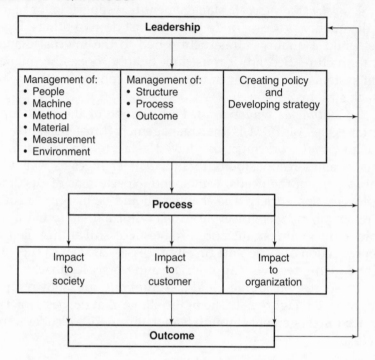

- Listen and then listen some more.
- Provide timely feedback.
- Support, direct, coach the employees.
- Communicate with everyone in the organization (vertically and horizontally).
- Apply the Plan – Do – Check (Study) – Act model as much as possible in everything within the organization.
- Reward and recognize the employees for teamwork, improvement, performance, and contribution to quality.

Once the leadership has been defined, then a policy, resources, and general management will guide the process, which, of course, is the real transformation of input into results based on the definitions of satisfaction of society, customer, and the organization.

TQM MODEL IN HEALTHCARE

Figure 2–2 shows the TQM model for healthcare. The major difference between this model and the one in Figure 2–1 is the fact that the customers in Figure 2–2 are much more convoluted than those in Figure 2–1. In addition, the requirements of outsiders, such as the government or the Joint Commission on Accreditation of Healthcare Organizations (JCAHO), present a somewhat different approach to quality. One may even suggest that TQM for healthcare is more prescriptive and appraisal oriented, primarily because of governmental regulations. After all, there are certain forms and procedures that have to be completed to make sure both the government and the JCAHO are satisfied. As a result, the left side of the model is shown with the quality of conformance, which by definition is more appraisal oriented. The perceived quality and the outcome of the model are the same in both models.

Application of the TQM Model

As already mentioned, TQM is doing the right thing right the first time, on time, all the time; always striving for improvement; and always attempting to satisfy the customer. This requires a focus on customer needs, people, system, and processes and a supportive cultural environment. In healthcare, the model may be used for the following processes throughout the organization:

Quality planning

- Identifying target market segments.
- Determining specific customer needs, wants, and expectations.
- Translating the customer needs into service and process requirements.
- Designing services and processes with the required characteristics. (Competitive benchmarking can assist in this part of the process.)

Quality control

- Measuring actual quality performance versus the design goals.

Conceptual Framework of the TQM Model in a Hospital

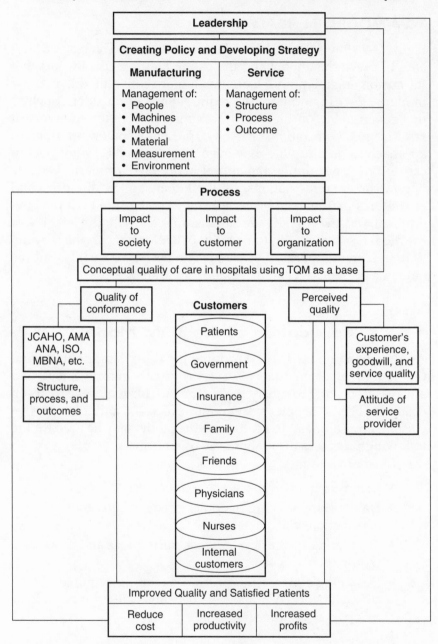

Note: AMA indicates American Medical Association; ANA, American Nurses Association; ISO, International Organization for Standardization; MBNA, Malcolm Baldrige National Award; JCAHO, Joint Commission on Accreditation of Healthcare Organizations.

- Diagnosing the cause of poor quality and initiating the required corrective steps.
- Establishing controls to maintain the gains.

Quality improvement

- Establishing a benchmarking process.
- Organizing a quality function deployment project.
- Providing the necessary resources.

It is imperative to note that the selected process:

1. Is strategic and proactive.
2. Competitively focuses on meeting customer needs as opposed to techniques of analysis.
3. Is comprehensive in terms of level and functions.
4. Manages in quality and not in terms of defect reduction.

R E F E R E N C E S

Bell, R. "Laying the Groundwork for a Smooth Transition to TQM." *Hospital Topics* 71, no. 1 (1993), pp. 23–26.

Greene, J. "TQM Means Big Investment, Multiple Year Wait for Results." *Modern Healthcare* 22, no. 41 (1992), p. 8.

Houghton, J. "TQM at Corning." *Health Systems Review* 25, no. 3 (1992), pp. 10–14.

Rooney, G. "TQM/CQI in Business and Healthcare." *AAOHN Journal* 40, no. 7 (1992), pp. 319–25.

Stamatis, D. H. *Total Quality Service*. Delray Beach, Fla.: St. Lucie Press, 1995.

CHAPTER 3

Teams

Teams are becoming the de facto operation in today's work environment, whether we deal in manufacturing, education, or healthcare. In this chapter an overview discussion of teams and self-directed teams will be offered. Furthermore, the relationship of teams and TQM will be discussed as it relates to the healthcare workplace.

DEFINITION OF TEAM

Webster's dictionary defines a team as follows:

team

A number of persons associated together in work or in an activity

Teams can also be referred to as a systems approach that leads us to develop a holistic understanding of the interrelated, interdependent quality of human interaction. Another definition of teams may be a view of all the interrelated elements (people) working together to achieve a common goal.

TYPES OF TEAMS

There are basically two types of teams. The part-time team involves people taking time away from their individual assignments to serve on task forces and committees. The full-time special-purpose team, also referred to as the composite team or cross-functional team, assigns the sole responsibilities of members in relation to the purpose(s) of the team. These teams usually include members from a cross section of the organization with a functional experience and knowledge (as in the case of different departments). More skill and knowledge than any one individual can provide are necessary to achieve the goals of a cross-functional team (Gooley 1993).

TEAM DEVELOPMENT

The success of a team depends on its development. It is vital that there is multifunctional and multidisciplinary involvement. Members may include customers, suppliers, marketers, attorneys, physicians, and nurses as well as accounting, financial, and purchasing personnel. A typical representation of the dynamics and makeup of a team is shown in Figure 3–1. There must be simultaneous full-time commitment. Simple cooperation and acceptance or responsibility on a part-time basis is not enough. The part-time team member is not really considered a team member at all.

It must be established and understood that any rewards will go to the team as a whole. Hence, evaluation will be based primarily on team performance. The "geographic" location of team members also is critical. They must have easy access to each other, in a sense "live together" or work together. Team members must also have access to any and all resources necessary to work toward accomplishment of the team's goal. The team structure must be established not under the principles of management but under those of leadership. Communication is a key to any team environment. It is essential that information and knowledge flow freely within the team and throughout the organization.

Once the team is established, it will go through two phases of interaction: formation and production. Formation is the initial period when the group begins to develop. People learn what roles they play. Often when individuals are selected to be a part of a team, there is no preassigned team leader. The best approach is to let a leader emerge from within the group. Other individuals will assume other roles accordingly. During the formation stage, group norms and rules are created. The function of the rules and norms

F I G U R E   3–1

Example of a Team Makeup

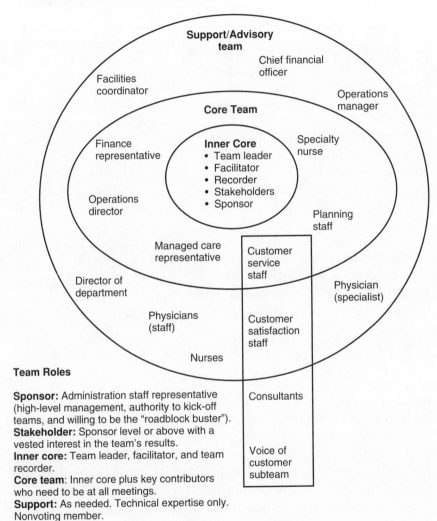

Team Roles

Sponsor: Administration staff representative (high-level management, authority to kick-off teams, and willing to be the "roadblock buster").
Stakeholder: Sponsor level or above with a vested interest in the team's results.
Inner core: Team leader, facilitator, and team recorder.
Core team: Inner core plus key contributors who need to be at all meetings.
Support: As needed. Technical expertise only. Nonvoting member.
Subteam: Miniteam, sponsored by main team. Must include at least one core member.

is to guide members' behaviors. Members need to understand and agree on the rules that guide their activities and their interactions. As a result, members develop a sense of equality within the group and a sense of belonging. The production phase is also referred to as the task-oriented phase, which is when the work gets accomplished.

TEAM EFFECTIVENESS

Factors that influence team effectiveness include the team members, the goals, and the environment. The team members must possess the necessary skills and must have the authority to make decisions. The goals must be clear and concise as well as operational (see Appendix B). The team must agree on the goals and take ownership of them. The total environment of the organization will dictate which elements are important and which ones will be encompassed for evaluation. For example, the organization's structure and culture have a great impact on the team's effectiveness. The policies and procedures and the systems (rewards and communication) also have an effect on the team.

Teams must manage how they work together and how they interact with the rest of the organization. An organizational structure conducive to teamwork would organize teams of people around tasks that require coordination and interdependence. The teams would have access to appropriate support groups.

ADVANTAGES AND DISADVANTAGES OF TEAMS

Advantages

In using teams, one of the greatest advantages is that communications between functions, people, and departments will improve and barriers will be eliminated. Team members have a feeling of belonging and contribution to the organization when they sense that an organization is open and does not work on the basis of intimidation. Many problems may be prevented in the inception stage because there is representation from many individuals with different points of view. These individuals may have diverse experiences, functions, and knowledge. Decisions are made by consensus, that is, participants must own their decisions as a team—one individual is not making a decision based on a hunch or opinion. The goals of the team are specific. Therefore, meetings are more efficient and are oriented to task improvement. An ability to get the job done exists even if it means circumventing the current system.

Motivation for change comes from within the team. Of course, there are economic benefits to teams. They create significant opportunities for leverage.

Disadvantages

The reward system for teams is sometimes inequitable among members. Often teams are created to "detour around" problems of dysfunctional organizations, instead of addressing them directly. Furthermore, many organizations assume they have developed a horizontal organization simply by renaming their departments as teams. Often there is a misunderstanding of, as well as resistance to, the concept and process of the team. The communication system within an organization can be set up to keep all team members informed of matters that affect them or to operate only through the established hierarchy, a process that may omit members of the team from participating effectively. This is common, particularly in cross-functional teams, in which some team members have not received important communications because they report to a leader who may not be in the appropriate distribution list for that communication.

RESOLVING TEAM CONFLICT

Tension or conflict often arises in a team-oriented environment. There are three types of tension that exist within teams: (1) primary, (2) secondary, and (3) tertiary. Primary tension usually occurs in the formation phase of the team. It comes out of the general concerns people have in any new environment. Any time people are moved out of their comfort zone, they need to identify what their new role is and to feel that they belong in their new environment. Secondary tensions evolve from disagreements in terms of ideas. They are usually prevalent in the operational (production) phase. Secondary tension is not necessarily negative; in fact, it can be considered productive when applied to the decision-making process. Tertiary tension comes from power struggles and can surface in either the formation or the operational phase. It is critical to the success of the team to overcome such conflict and proceed to obtain the universal goals.

There are seven key actions to take to resolve team tensions or conflict:

1. Promptly make the people involved aware of how their conflict is affecting the team's performance. The team members need to understand why "their business" is the team's business. Linking the conflict's impact on the team is the most direct, appropriate, and credible way to address team conflict. Keeping everyone's attention on the work-related problem—not the personalities involved—can help make it clear why it is important to resolve the conflict. Focus on the situation, issue, or behavior, not on the individual. To illustrate the point, explain the specific performance measures that reveal the problem, such as schedule slippage, cost overruns, or reduced output.

2. Set up a joint problem-solving approach, with the entire team, to resolve the conflict. This will give everyone an opportunity to present his or her side of an issue. Since everyone will need to support the final solution, it is sensible to include them in the problem-solving process. This action of the team will also strengthen the ownership of the solution.

3. Ask the individuals involved in the conflict to present their viewpoints objectively. Unless each party involved has the opportunity to present his or her side, the result may be disastrous. More resentment and misunderstanding may surface. While an individual is presenting, prevent any interruptions by others, keep the discussion focused on the problem, and curtail any blaming.

4. Obtain agreement on the problem that needs to be solved. Often people will deny that a problem exists or will jump to solutions before a problem is clarified. This hinders the effectiveness of addressing the true problem.

5. Each team member is responsible for generating possible solutions. Once again, involvement evokes ownership.

6. Each team member must commit to focus on conflict resolution. Once the alternative solutions have been identified, the best solution or combination of solutions must be agreed on. Assign individual responsibilities accordingly.

7. Summarize what has been discussed. Plan to meet soon to review the progress of the conflict resolution. It is important to understand that every team member encounters conflict at some time or another. Each time conflict is addressed and people work together for a solution, a collaborative and initiative-based approach becomes established for the team to follow. People will learn how to work out difficulties independently, before conflicts enlarge and demand too much of the team's attention.

REENGINEERING THE STRUCTURE

With the environment and technology ever changing and the spread of information technology and computer networks, the dismantling of hierarchy is with us. It is important that organizations transform themselves radically to survive and become more competitive. One way organizations are surmounting these extenuating circumstances is to reengineer or revolutionize the organization, that is, to undergo a radical or complete change in the organization's structure. Recently, self-managed, cross-functional teams have become the basis for revolutionizing organizations.

Too many layers of management hinder the decision-making process. They lead to high coordination and overhead costs. They develop functional barriers. And they result in lack of communication or miscommunication. Layers of management need to be removed and employees need to be empowered. Processes have to be thought out and redefined to be effective and current. Jobs and tasks also must reflect these changes. Management of the organization must be horizontal rather than vertical. This largely eliminates both hierarchical and functional boundaries. For reengineering to work it is essential that everyone in the organization works together in cross-functional teams that perform core processes. This cooperation between employees and management will make the teams the main building blocks of the reorganization process.

TEAM PROBLEM SOLVING
AND PROCESS IMPROVEMENT

The question always comes up in discussing TQM and process improvement, Why a team approach? Indeed a simple question, but a very powerful one. So, let us look at it from a closer perspective. Since the middle 1970s we have been bombarded with the concept of employee involvement (EI), quality circles (QC), quality of work life (QWL), and so on. The goal of these programs has been to give people increased influence over and responsibility for their own work. In recent years one of the major routes to achieving this goal has been the creation of problem-solving teams. Employees who are appropriately trained meet regularly to identify and solve work-related problems.

As the early results of problem-solving teams started to come in, managers realized that they had a vast, untapped potential in their employees' minds. Successful companies worldwide credit much of their success to the widespread use of employee teams to generate improvement in all departments and at all levels. Managers finally recognized that the people closest to the task are the most qualified to talk about and improve their work environments.

Today, to remain competitive, it is essential to make effective use of all the talents that our labor force has to offer, both physical and mental. We need to offer the opportunity to participate in the decision making and problem solving that affect them. This will ensure an ownership to the corrective action or solution put into place. To be effective, however, we need to provide employees with appropriate and applicable training and with challenging activities to keep their minds fully utilized.

Finally, the most effective, proven problem-solving and process improvement methods and tools lend themselves best to a team approach. They operate under the rubric of synergy, which tells us that a team will invariably generate more problems, more causes, and more solutions than any one individual can. No one person has all the knowledge about processes, products, and services plus the special skills and experience required for optimal problem solving.

When we talk about teams in the quest of quality we differentiate the terms *local* and *cross-functional*. Local or department improvement teams are composed of all the members of a department. These employees typically work in close proximity, experience common problems, and form a natural work group. Their purpose is to provide a focus and a means for all employees to contribute to an ongoing activity aimed at improving the quality and productivity levels of the department. On the other hand, cross-functional teams, also called process action teams or process improvement teams, are created to continuously improve quality, reduce waste, and improve productivity of a process that crosses many departmental lines. This type of team is made up of experienced, skilled problem solvers from all departments involved in and affected by the process.

Guidelines for Effective Team Problem Solving and Process Improvement

For a team to function successfully, it requires the following:

- A team charter, which specifies the team's purpose and enumerates the team's duties and responsibilities.
- Selection of the proper team makeup.
- Selection of an effective team leader and team coordinator (facilitator).
- Knowledge of the organization's mission, goals, and objectives.
- Team building (learning to work together as a team).
- Adequate training in problem solving and process improvement methods and tools.
- Guidelines and ground rules for holding effective meetings and making decisions.
- An adequate meeting place with needed support services, such as typing, word processing, computer help, and copying access to appropriate information.
- Use of meeting agendas and minutes.
- Liberal credit and recognition for team successes.

SELF-DIRECTED WORK TEAMS

Never before in the history of the workplace has the concept of teamwork been more important to the functions of successful organizations. With the rapid social, technological, and informational changes that are occurring, our society is faced with stresses never before encountered. Our organizations are more competitive. No longer can we depend on a few peak performances or on a few performers to rise to the top to lead. If we are to survive, we must figure out ways to tap into the creativity and potential of people at all levels (Blanchard, Carew, and Carew, 1990). It is becoming increasingly clear that organizational responses such as new product and service development, cross-functional projects, and technology deployment, as well as initiatives like TQM, require a flexible and empowered workforce. Put more succinctly, without levels of empowerment, projects and programs will not deliver the promised results. Speed, quality, productivity, and new services come from people, not programs.

Let us then look at the issue of empowerment. What is it?

empowerment

A function of four characteristics always working in tandem: authority, responsibility (accountability), resources, and information

To be empowered, employees need formal authority and all the resources (budget, time, equipment, training, etc.) necessary to do something with the new acquired authority. They also need timely, accurate, and current information to make good decisions. Finally, they need a personal sense of accountability for the work.

Empowerment gives people greater control over their own destiny. There are various degrees of empowerment. Employee involvement with lower empowerment techniques such as selected employee input on projects are on one end of the scale, ongoing employee task forces and quality vision are in the middle of the scale, and higher empowerment processes such as self-directed work teams (SDWTs) are on the other end of the scale. A typical representation may look like the following:

Employee suggestions	Quality vision	SDWTs

Low ⟵————————————————⟶ High

What Are Self-Directed Teams?

A slightly modified version of the definition of an SDWT used by the Association for Quality and Participation is as follows:

self-directed work team

A group of employees who have day-to-day responsibility for managing themselves and the work they do with a minimum of direct supervision

Members of self-directed teams typically handle job assignments, plan and schedule related decisions, and take action on problems.

Self-directed teams work. They have been around as early as the 1960s. They also get results. SDWTs (everything else being equal) get better results than their traditional counterparts. In a review cited by Fisher (1993) of organizations that had transitioned from traditional work systems to SDWTs in seven countries, J. Cotter, a prominent sociotechnical system consultant, found that 93 percent of the teams improved productivity, 86 percent decreased operating costs, 86 percent improved quality, and 70 percent created better employee attitudes. Fisher also reported that these findings were confirmed with results from the following companies: Digital Equipment Co., Tektronix, Mead, TRW, James River, Procter & Gamble, Martin Marietta, General Electric, ESSO, American Transtech, and others.

In healthcare, from my experience, positive results have been substantiated in Henry Ford Hospital, University of Michigan Medical Center, St. Claire Hospital, and other facilities. In all these examples, self-directed work teams frequently have outperformed comparable traditional operations. Unlike a number of other corporate initiatives that have promised fire but delivered mostly smoke, SDWTs have often improved many of the key organizational measures by 30 to 50 percent.

Of course, SDWTs do not always get results. When they do not get positive results, one of the strongest possibilities for the failure is that the SDWT was not given appropriate and applicable authority and responsibility within its environment. In other words, the team was not appropriately empowered.

Within healthcare, SDWTs may be used in a variety of functions and at various levels. The reason for this flexibility is the fact that SDWTs operate in their daily functions free from the old concept of the division of labor. As a result of this freedom, they require a minimal amount (if any) of direct supervision. This is in total contrast to the old span of control of traditional management where it was typical for 10 to 15 employees to report to one supervisor (Odiorne 1991). With SDWTs this traditional approach to management is refuted. It is not unusual for one layer of management to be eliminated and the span of control to be 70 to 80 employees per supervisor.

Odiorne (1991) has identified five reasons why the trend in all types of organizations is toward SDWTs. They are presented here, somewhat modified:

1. The old division of labor idea, with one order giver supervising 10 order takers, has proved to be a source of apathy, anger, and alienation to the people at the bottom. This, in turn, leads to poor quality, low productivity, and dissatisfied customers.

2. Our economy has shifted from being production centered to service centered. This means more white-collar workers have higher level expectations from their jobs than do the traditional blue-collar workers. They expect to be consulted, not bossed. When they are not consulted, they become disappointed, frustrated, angry, and apathetic.

3. The best service organizations are pushing the team concept for service down lower in the organization. Good service means forming teams that work as a unit and that accomplish a completed task as defined. Service by self-managed teams is based on creative problem solving and initiative. Such an approach can bring about renewal and result in stimulating and invigorating organizations.

4. Empowerment is an important element of the new management style. This suggests a new kind of organizational structure, with decisions being made by people who are truly empowered to make them free from a bureaucratic leadership emanating from the top.

5. Marketing has changed from the individual purchasing agent to team buying and team selling. The selling organization is a customer problem-solving team, not just a solo salesperson.

Another reason for the trend in using SDWTs is technology. Technology—especially in healthcare—facilitates group decision making, problem solving, information gathering, and information assessing. Technology can also provide some substitutes for the information passing and coordination role of the traditional hierarchy. This allows teams to be directed by the work and the information rather than by managers. This change also implies that the style of managing will have to change, which may result in some resistance (Hicks and Bono 1990). The resistance may take the form of at least the following:

1. Supervisors and middle managers see participative management as a watering down of their authority and power.
2. Moving too fast in making sweeping changes leads to foot dragging, hesitancy, and lower productivity and quality.
3. People who are used to autocratic leadership have become accustomed to taking and following orders issued by the boss and are uncomfortable with a new approach.
4. Teams of 15 or so have a tendency to split into smaller interest groups. The fact that there are pitfalls that exist does not mean the concept is flawed or unworkable.

How do we start SDWTs in the workplace? Wellins (1992) and Stamatis (1994) have proposed the following steps:

1. Appropriate training of upper management in the concept of SDWT.

2. Perform a readiness assessment to determine the current culture of the organization.

3. Communicate the organization's vision and values as they relate to teams and the issue of empowerment. Management must have a clear picture of where the company is heading and how the concept of self-direction ties in with existing missions and cultural values.

4. Take your organization through a workplace redesign, always emphasizing the core processes. This process requires looking at your existing work through work flow diagrams, job design layout, and procedures. It will also require an investigation of the organization's overall system for compatibility through structure, evaluation policies, compensation, training, and so on.

5. Implement into the work environment. This should be based on a sound change process, such as open communication, leadership support, and training.

All SDWTs are dynamic, complex, ever changing, living systems that develop their own patterns of behavior. However, there are four basic stages that seem to be common to all SDWTs: orientation, dissatisfaction, resolution, and operation.

Stages of SDWTs

1. *Orientation.* The orientation stage is when the individuals come together for the first time. Some characteristics of this stage are:

- High expectations.
- Feelings of anxiety: Where do I fit? What is expected of me?
- Testing the situation.
- Need to find one's place and secure it.

At this stage the team leader generally uses high directive behavior (directing) to clarify the mission, set roles and goals, and define tasks.

2. *Dissatisfaction.* The dissatisfaction stage finds the group in limbo and there is no development. Quite often in this stage we find the team leader acting as a facilitator, assisting the team in the right direction and motivating them to express their thoughts and opinions. The team leader also acts as a coach for the team members to improve skills, methods, approaches, and so on at this problem development or dissatisfaction stage. Some of the characteristics of this stage are:

- A discrepancy between "hope" and "reality."
- Dissatisfaction with dependence on authority.
- Frustration and anger around goals, tasks, and action plans.
- Feelings of incompetence and confusion.
- Negative reaction toward leaders and other members.
- Competition for power and/or attention.
- Experiencing polarities—dependence or counterdependence.

3. *Resolution.* The resolution stage is the stage at which the team comes around to openly discuss disagreements without hard feelings toward each other. The team starts to work together as a team. The role of the team leader is that of a supporter on everything the team needs. In a few instances the team leader will act as a director. Some of the characteristics of this stage are:

- Decreasing dissatisfaction.
- Resolution of discrepancies between expectation and reality.
- Resolution of polarities and animosities.
- Development of harmony, trust, support, and respect.
- Development of self-esteem and confidence.
- Increase in openness and giving feedback.
- Shared responsibility and control.
- Use of team language: "we" instead of "I."

4. *Operation* (production). The operational stage is when the group achieves normal enthusiastic behavior as they approach the task at hand. The team works together, sharing information and proposing ideas. The team moves as a unit, with different people taking leadership at different times. The team leader at this stage seems to have little impact. In fact, usually, the team leader becomes one of the team members, with no special privileges or accolades.

Selection of Team Participants

Wellins (1992) has identified four major features for the selection process of the SDWT members. They are:

1. The selection system must be accurate in identifying the candidates who are likely to succeed in the new organizational structure.
2. The system of selection must be legally defensible.
3. Selection must be perceived as fair. Candidates should believe that they are treated in a just manner and that the system has accurately assessed their potential for performing the jobs in question.
4. The selection system must be efficient.

When selecting team participants, management and certainly the personnel department should be involved. Once the team has been selected, the targets should be defined based on the expected performance. The requirements for membership include but are not limited to knowledge in teamwork, problem identification and solution, ability to learn, communication, initiative, work standards, coaching and training, job motivation, technical ability and work tempo (ability to work at a relatively fast and constant speed).

When selecting the team leader, both management and the personnel department should be looking at several additional requirements beyond the requirements for membership. A team leader must have individual and team leadership talent, knowledge about quality issues, good judgment, ability to delegate, initiative, enthusiasm, and coaching skills.

Once the selection process has been completed, the team is ready for setting the ground rules of the team. What follows is a cursory summary of this process. (Additional information on goals may be found in Appendix B.)

Ground Rules of Work Teams

Successful SDWTs have certain ground rules to which they must adhere. Glassman (1992) and Stamatis (1994, 1995) have identified the following rules:

1. The team atmosphere should be nonthreatening.
2. Cooperation and teamwork should be encouraged.
3. The primary goal is to accomplish team goals.
4. Every member must participate and contribute.
5. Technical leadership and follower roles should not be monopolized.
6. Work experience in the team environment should be enjoyable and pleasant.
7. Feedback and evaluation should be accepted and encouraged.

Development of the Team

Development of an SDWT involves time and skill from both management and team participants. A typical development is in the areas of diagnostics, adaptability, empowerment, and training.

Diagnostics

All team participants must, in no uncertain terms, be able to diagnose the process under consideration. They must be familiar with the process itself as well as with which approach will expedite a solution to the problem.

Adaptability

All team participants must learn to work within the system. They must learn to adapt to different situations. If drastic changes are about to be introduced, they have to prepare the personnel involved for those changes.

Empowerment

All team participants must be empowered to do what has to be done without fear of incriminating themselves, without fear of retaliation, without fear of the administration getting even with them, without fear of being labeled a troublemaker, without fear of being labeled as having a negative attitude, without fear of being named an instigator, and so on. True empowerment will be demonstrated with appropriate and applicable authority and responsibility to do what has to be done to get the job done within the scope of the team.

Training

All participants must be trained and continue to be trained in a just-as-needed fashion. The initial minimum training ought to cover items, such as communication and participation dynamics, decision making, leadership roles, goal setting, team dynamics, conflict resolution, and problem solving. As the team grows and needs more specific training, that training may be provided on a just-as-needed basis. Some just-as-needed training may be benchmarking, needs assessment training, quality function deployment, and design of experiments.

HEALTHCARE AND TEAMS

Across the United States individual organizations within the healthcare industry are focusing on strengthening their competitive positions and substantially increasing their profits. To do that, individual organizations are entering the world of continuous improvement. Continuous improvement aims to capture immediate improvement opportunities, build the skills and confidence that will enable the organization to identify and capture opportunities on an ongoing basis, and instill a readiness in employees to embrace continuous change.

To be successful in such an undertaking, continuous improvement must become *the central* thinking of management. It starts with the formation of teams and continues with institutionalizing the knowledge gained, to improve even further. Teams may contribute in the following areas:

- Measuring performance, including productivity, customer service, and quality.
- Setting concrete goals at all organizational levels, for both productivity and customer satisfaction.
- Strengthening accountability for results (not activities).
- Focusing on customer satisfaction (both internal and external).
- Building continuous improvement into the core process, rather than treating the improvement as a supplement to core management processes.

The primary responsibility for change remains with line managers; however, they can and should be supplemented with teams to facilitate the transfer of knowledge and skills across like departments. This, of course, will materialize with appropriate training provided to management and nonmanagement employees alike.

Teams should be the primary vehicle for reaching all the continuous improvement objectives. Specific objectives may take the form of the following:

Deliver measurable performance improvements while trying new ways of managing excitement and commitment within the organization.

- Identify a specific goal within a specified time.
- Capitalize on the empowerment and move forward with continuous improvement thinking.
- Use data for your analysis and challenge old paradigms.

- Understand the changes and their implication to both your own organization and to your customer.

Develop a standard method and a set of tools with which the team can identify and capture the ongoing activities and improvements.

- One of the most basic methods is the Plan-Do-Check (Study)-Act known as the PDCA cycle.
- The methodology and basic tools taught while teams are in the organizational stage are:

Identification stage:

- Brainstorming
- Process flow
- Cause-and-effect diagram

Analysis stage:

- Pareto chart
- Histogram
- Run chart
- Check sheet
- Scatter diagram

Plan stage:

- Work plan
- Quality plan

Develop a plan that goes *beyond* achieving the initial goals.

- Identify how the initial process changes will be implemented in the specific departments.
- Identify which data need to be tracked and the frequency of the data, and analyze to ensure performance gains.
- Identify which new areas would be worth exploring.

The essence of the approach is to prepare the organization for continuous improvement. Formation of teams will not only achieve an immediate performance gain but also build in their participants the skills and readiness to achieve further gains. It must be emphasized that these are not ad hoc teams or one-time teams. These are perpetual teams that move from a problem (opportunity) to a different problem (opportunity), with a specific goal to resolve that particular problem (opportunity) with a positive result.

Sometimes in healthcare the terms *breakthrough team* or *affinity team* surface, and they need to be explained. A breakthrough team is a multidisciplinary and cross-functional team that looks at problems (opportunities) in the work environment. Team members set goals to either improve the process or to eliminate the problem completely. They do that through a systematic problem-solving approach under a Kaizen (incremental) system or through revolutionary change in the process.

On the other hand, an affinity team is a cross-functional team whose primary purpose is to ensure the efficient transfer of knowledge, skills, and better practices throughout a particular department. For example, a health provider operates four different facilities, each of which has separate radiology (x-ray) departments. Each one of these departments operates independently of each other, with its own structure, policy, and procedures. The continuous improvement fever has caught on in this health provider, and corporate management has decided to form teams for improvement. The result of an affinity team will be x-ray departments that share their knowledge, skills, and practices with each other and that likely will form standardized practices.

The specific responsibilities of an affinity team may include the following:

- Share knowledge around a specific system, including better practices, policies, and ideas.
- Define and disseminate standard productivity and quality measures that are consistently used across the organization.
- Identify and sponsor initiatives that capture opportunities beyond the scope of individual areas.
- Mandate a limited number of standards that require uniformity across the system.

To reinforce continuous improvement, training and coaching skills should be developed for all employees who will actively participate in the team development and implementation. Some of the concerns in the training curriculum for supervisors and managers are:

- How to think of their units as profit cost centers, while at the same time realizing that their success may depend on adjacent or totally independent departments.
- How to set stretching goals each year for productivity, quality, and customer service.
- How to measure performance regularly and how to communicate the performance results to their entire departments.
- How to use analytical tools to solve problems and meet specific goals.
- How to reasonably demand accountability from employees.
- How to generate an appropriate and applicable budget.
- How to allocate appropriate funds and time for specific projects.

Concerns in training also exist for team leaders and facilitators. Fundamentally the team leader or the facilitator uses the leadership role to develop skills and confidence in others and to create an attitude of becoming a continuously improving organization. This facilitator may be called the ambassador for the project. Furthermore, the team leader can also be the conduit for the managers and supervisors to help make key changes in work practices. Some training recommendations for the team leader and facilitator are:

- How to challenge the team's thinking and help them conduct thorough analyses.
- How to help or coach the team members to become better problem solvers.
- How to push—without being a dictator—for real wins, that is, when a team meets its goal using a process that leads to continuous improvement, not just a one-shot gain.
- How to ensure that improvements are sustainable, to institutionalize the team's gains.
- How to encourage the team to take on barriers to change.
- How to motivate team members from an intrinsic point of view as opposed to an extrinsic point of view.
- How to build the team's confidence.

REFERENCES

Blanchard, K.; D. Carew; and E. Carew. *The One Minute Manager, Builds High Performing Teams.* New York: William Morrow, 1990.

Buchoholz, S., and T. Roth. *Creating the High Performance Team.* New York: John Wiley & Sons, 1987.

Dyer, W. G. *Team Building.* 2d ed. Reading, Mass.: Addison-Wesley, 1987.

Fisher, F. *Leading Self Directed Work Teams.* New York: McGraw-Hill, 1993.

Glassman, E. "Self Directed Team Building without a Consultant." *Supervisory Management,* March 1992, pp. 6–7.

Gooley, T. B. "Team Spirit." *Traffic Management,* September 1993, pp. 14–16.

Hicks, R. F., and D. Bono. *Self Managed Teams.* Los Altos, Calif.: Crisp Publications, 1990.

Odiorne, G. S. "The New Breed of Supervisor: Leaders in Self Managed Work Teams." *Supervision,* August 1991, pp. 14–17.

Stamatis, D. H. *Teams and SDWT.* Southgate, Mich.: Contemporary Consultants, 1994.

———. *Total Quality Service.* Delray Beach, Fla.: St. Lucie Press, 1995.

"Tips for Training." *Training,* February 1994, p. 14.

Wellins, R. S. "Building a Self Directed Work Team." *Training and Development,* December 1992, pp. 24–28.

CHAPTER 4

Data Collection
and Analysis

Much has been said about measurement in the field of quality. Measurement is so important that it is one of the principles of Deming's philosophy and of total quality management. In the quality profession we live and die by some form of number evaluation from the process, supplier, customer, and so on. It is so common that we all have been conditioned to think of data-driven organizations. The problem is, how do we handle data, and what do we do with the data after collection? In this chapter we will address the following questions:

How do you make sure that the appropriate data have been collected?

How do you apply the correct statistical test?

What is significance anyway?

It has been said that statistics is the art of lying by means of figures. If that is the case, how do we get to the statistics and what, if any, is their significance? To answer this simple question, we must first understand the concept of data and then understand the preparation and analysis of data.

DATA CONCEPTS

datum

Any single observation about a specified characteristic of interest

Datum is the basic unit of the quality staffperson's raw material. Any collection of observations about one or more characteristics of interest for one or more elementary units is called a data set. A data set is said to be univariate, bivariate, or multivariate depending on whether it contains information on one variable, two variables, or more than two variables (Hays 1981).

The set of all possible observations about a specific characteristic of interest is called a population or universe. It is important to note that when we speak of population or universe, by definition, we speak of *all possible* observations about a variable. Any subset (portion) of the population or universe is called a sample.

Caution should be exercised in the use of these terms because a population or sample depends entirely on how the question is raised. A sample may be a population, and a population may be a sample. For example, a hospital laboratory had to retest 25 blood tests. On the other hand, the regional lab industry in the same period had to retest 1,500 blood tests. If the laboratory wants to analyze the 25 tests only, the 25 tests become the population of this study. If, however, the laboratory wants to analyze and compare the 25 tests with the 1,500 tests, the 25 tests are a sample of all the blood tests in that region.

In addition to the sample versus population concern, when addressing the issue of data, invariably one will notice that any given characteristic of interest can differ in kind or in degree among various elementary units. A variable that is normally expressed numerically because it differs in kind rather than degree is called a qualitative variable. Qualitative variables can be dichotomous or multinominal. Dichotomous qualitative variables are also called attribute or categorical variables because they are of two categories. Examples are: Go/no go, male/female, good/bad, and on/off. Multinominal qualitative variables can be made in more than two categories. Examples are: job titles, types of business, and colors (Hays 1981; Becker and Harnett 1987; Freund and Williams 1972).

A variable that is normally expressed numerically because it differs in degree rather than kind is called a quantitative variable. Quantitative variables can be discrete or continuous. Observations about discrete quantitative variables can assume values only at specific points on a scale of values, with gaps between them. Examples are: patients waiting in the emergency room and certain prescription drugs in inventory.

Observations about continuous quantitative variables can, in contrast, assume values at all points on a scale of values, with no breaks or gaps between them. Examples are: weight, time, temperature, pressure, and volume. No matter how close two values are to each other, *it is always possible* for a more precise device to find another value between them (Hays 1981; Mansfield 1983; Kerlinger 1973).

The distinction between qualitative and quantitative variables is visually obvious. The observations about one type of variable are recorded in words; those about the other type, in numbers. Yet the distinction can be blurred. Quantitative variables can be converted into seemingly qualitative ones and the opposite is also true. For example, when we speak of high or low temperature or pressure, we have taken a quantitative (measurable) variable and transformed it to an attribute (subjective) variable. When this coding takes place, information is lost in the process. Conversely, it is not uncommon to code attribute variables with numerical values, for example, "good" as 1 and "bad" as 0.

TYPES OF DATA

The assignment of numbers or values to characteristics that are being observed—which is measurement—can yield four types of data of increasing sophistication. It can produce nominal, ordinal, interval, or ratio data. Different statistical concepts and techniques are appropriately applied to each type. For the details of the selection process, see Figures 4–1, 4–2, and 4–3.

The weakest level of measurement produces nominal data, which are numbers that merely name or label differences in kind and thus can serve the purpose of classifying observations about qualitative variables into mutually exclusive groups. No mathematical operations are possible except counting.

The next level of measurement produces ordinal data, which are numbers that, by their size, order or rank observations on the basis of importance, while intervals between those numbers are meaningless. Again, no arithmetic operations are possible.

In the third level of sophistication are the interval data that

FIGURE 4–1

The Road Map to Statistical Analysis with Nominal Data

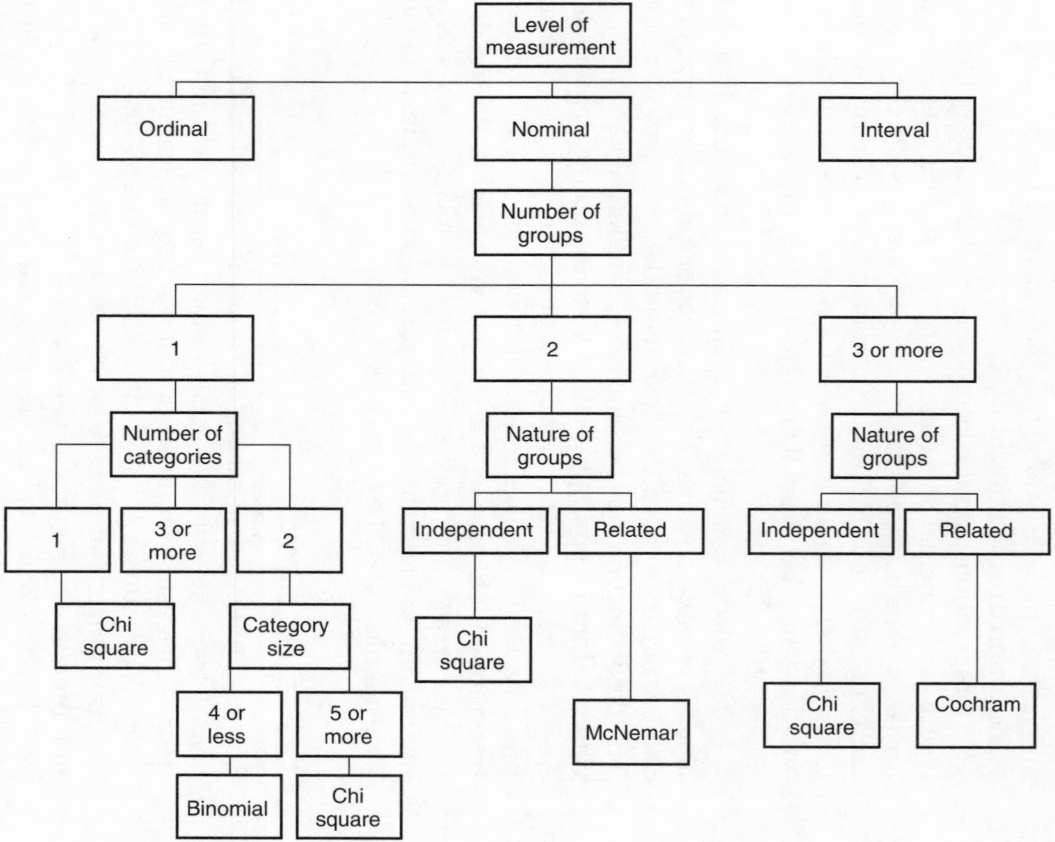

F I G U R E   4–2

The Road Map to Statistical Analysis with Ordinal Data

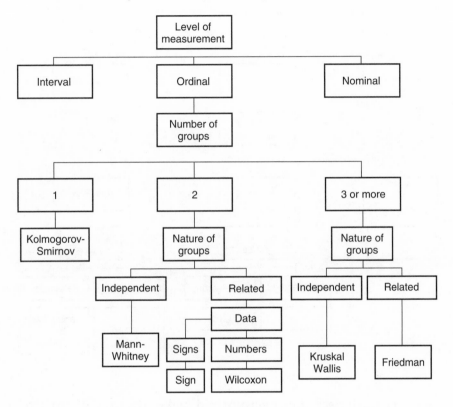

permit at least addition and subtraction. Interval data are numbers that, by their size, rank observations in order of importance and between which intervals or distances are comparable, while their ratios are meaningless. This kind of data possesses no meaningful origin and thus by a given definition establishes the zero point as well as equally arbitrary intervals between numbers. The Likert-type evaluation scale is an example of such data.

The most useful type of data is the ratio data, which are numbers that, by their size, rank observations in order of importance and between which intervals and ratios are meaningful. All types of arithmetic operations are possible because these numbers have a natural or a "true" zero point that denotes the complete absence

F I G U R E   4–3

The Road Map to Statistical Analysis with Internal Data

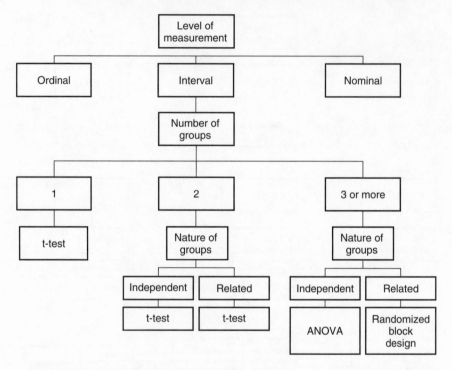

of the characteristic they measure and makes the ratio of any two such numbers independent of the unit measurement. Examples of such data are temperature, volume, and weight.

DATA COLLECTION

Data can be gathered in different forms. First, however, the purpose of the data must be determined. Only then can a decision be made as to which kind of data would best serve the purpose. There can be many purposes for collecting data in the world of quality. Some common purposes are Deming (1966) and Sharp (1979):

   1. Understanding of the actual situation. Data are collected to check the extent of the current process.

   2. Analysis. Data are collected to perform statistical analysis for a historical perspective of the process and/or future behavior of the same process.

3. Process control. After investigating product quality, data can be used to determine whether the process is normal. In this case, control charts are used in the evaluatior. and action is taken on the basis of these data.

4. Regulation. These data are used as the basis for regulating the process based on a previously set goal.

5. Acceptance or rejection. This form of data is used to approve or reject parts and/or products after inspection. There are two methods: (a) total inspection and (b) sampling. On the basis of the information obtained, a decision can be made as to what to do with the parts or products.

It is imperative that the purpose of data collection is not to put everything into neat figures but to provide a basis for action. The data may be in any form but generally are divided into the measurement data and the countable (attribute) data.

Once the purpose of the data has been defined, data can be generated by conducting a survey or by performing an experiment. A survey or observational study is the collection of data from basic units without exercising any particular control over factors that may make these units different from one another and that may therefore affect the characteristic of interest being observed. An experiment, on the other hand, involves the collection of data from basic units, while exercising control over some or all factors that may make these units different from one another and that may therefore affect the characteristic of interest being observed.

SAMPLING DATA

As mentioned earlier, data are gathered before working on problems to provide information to ensure that everything is within allowable tolerances and under control. Data can also be analyzed when things go out of control to find out what went wrong. Ideally, 100 percent of the given output would be checked for problems. However, this is not usually feasible because of time and cost considerations. Representative data can be acquired by closely sampling the given output. This allows the use of smaller numbers, for generalization to the entire population (output). There are three types of samples used in all forms of statistical analysis:

1. *Convenience sample.* When expediency is of primary concern as a consequence, a not so representative sample may be selected.

2. *Judgment sample.* A personal judgment is used for the selection of the sample based on some previous experience. Although used in the field of quality, caution should be exercised because of inherent biases by the selector of the sample.

3. *Random or probability sample.* Unrepresentativeness is not one of the characteristics of a random sample. Rather, it is a subset of a population, chosen by a random process that gives each unit of that population a known positive *but not necessarily equal* chance to be selected. If properly executed the random selection process allows no discretion to the experimenter as to which particular units in the population enter the sample. This form of sampling maximizes the chance of making valid inferences about the totality from which it is drawn.

There are four types of random sampling:

1. *Simple.* A simple random sample is a subset of a population chosen in such a fashion that every possible subset of like size has an equal chance of being selected. Here be cautioned in that the implication of each individual unit of the population has an equal chance of being selected, but the converse is not true, that is, giving each individual unit an equal chance of being selected does not assure every possible subset of like size of having an equal chance.

2. *Systematic.* A systematic random sample is a subset of a population chosen by randomly selecting one of the first elements and then inducing every *ith* element thereafter. In this procedure the *i* is determined by dividing the population size, N, by the desired sample size, n.

3. *Stratified.* A stratified random sample is a subset of a population chosen by taking separate (simple or systematic) random samples from every stratum in the population, often in such a way that the sizes of the separate samples vary with the importance of the different strata.

4. *Clustered.* A clustered random sample is a subset of a population, chosen by taking separate censuses in a randomly chosen subset of geographically distinct clusters.

ERRORS IN DATA

The process of gathering information is one of collecting and filtering data. The ultimate solution is a combination of good information at all levels, structures that size the decision-making process, and personal reconnaissance on the part of the decision maker at each level.

Statistics, even when most accurate, can never be the complete substitute for an in-depth knowledge of the situation of collecting, filtering, and analyzing data. Deming (1986) addresses this issue when he points out that there is a difference between visible and invisible numbers. He comments that some managers look only at the visible numbers, "but the visible numbers tell them so little. They know nothing of the invisible numbers. Who can put a price on a satisfied customer, and who can figure out the cost of a dissatisfied customer?"

All large samples have two kinds of errors. The first is a random error or chance error or sampling error. This error is the difference between the value of a variable obtained by taking a single random sample and the value obtained by taking the population. The second error is the systematic error or bias or nonsampling and is the difference between the value of a variable obtained by taking the population and the true value. Another way of explaining these errors is by thinking of sampling error as the reliability of data and nonsampling as the validity of the data.

Reliability is a concept like repeatability. If you keep repeating, in all executionary details, there is a probability that your sample will have an operating range. Furthermore, it will have a degree of stability, based on that operating range. Note that this has nothing to do with how accurate your sample was. This is a trap that most practitioners fall into and they are justified with what is called confidence statement or statistical significance. To speak of 90, 95, or even 99 percent confidence is an issue of limited value in management, knowing that findings of a particular sample would probably be similar to those of a second and/or third sample if they were identically conducted. Such knowledge begs the issue of whether the sample method was good in the first place. Statements of statistical significance beg the issue of data validity and hence the sample's usefulness.

One can hardly list all possible types of nonsampling error, all the ways that a sample can yield misleading data, and all sources of invalid information about a target process. Only a few biases are listed here, by stage:

Planning Stage

- Selection bias is a systematic tendency to favor the inclusion in a sample of selected basic units with particular characteristics while excluding other units with other characteristics.
- Response bias is a tendency for selection of a sample to be wrong in some systematic way.

Collection Stage

- Selection bias is apt to enter the sample when experimenters are instructed to select, within broad guidelines, the particular characteristics that they will sample.
- Response bias can arise for a number of reasons during data collection. Both the experimenter and the process may be at fault.
- Nonresponse bias may arise when no legitimate data are available from the sample.

Processing Stage

The emergence of bias during data collection can conceivably be minimized by the careful design of the sample. Nevertheless, bias can enter even at the data processing stage. People who code, edit, keypunch, tabulate, print, and otherwise manipulate data have many opportunities for making noncanceling errors. One of the major concerns in the quality area is the issue of data "outliers" or "wild values." We have a tendency to eliminate unbelievable data (high, low, or just different from the majority) or to substitute zero for a "no value" and vice versa.

CONTROL OF THE DATA

To optimize the results of your data, the following may be considered.

   1. Weighting sample data. It is a technique nothing more than

the multiplication of sample observations by one or more factors to increase or decrease the emphasis that will be given to the observation. The troublesome aspect of weighting is related to the selection or calculation of the weighting factors. The specifications of the weighting scheme must be defined in terms of our overall objective. What is the purpose of weighting? In most cases, the obvious answer is that we would like our sample data to be representative of the population. The immediate follow-up to the first question is another: In what ways are the data to be representative of the population? The answer to this question should lead us to select an appropriate technique.

2. Beware of the *homing pigeon* syndrome. This is where you become completely dependent for data on the incoming paper flow; you lose the interactive process and find out only what the sender wants you to know.

3. Reports and data required from the bottom up must be balanced by data interchange from the top down. The same old questions get the same old answers. If the system does not allow for an interchange in the data flow process, you will soon find yourself asking the wrong questions, at which point the answers do not matter.

4. Have an appropriate sample for the specific project. It is imperative that we have the correct sample plan figured out before we begin experimenting. It is beyond the focus of this book to discuss the mathematical calculations for sampling. However, any statistics book may be of help.

5. Missing data. It is one of the most common problems in the field of quality. We all have a tendency to fill in the blanks of missing data. When we as experimenters do that, it is the worst possible alternative. The reasons for this are that (*a*) we do not really know the outcome; therefore, we are guessing and (*b*) we are forcing a distribution of our data that is not really representative of what we are studying. If we do have missing data—for whatever reason—treat it as such. In case of computer use, most software programs have a built-in command for handling the missing data. The identification of missing data conventionally is noted as a dot ("*.*").

6. Types of errors. When you have collected the data, there have been several assumptions about the data and its significance.

One of the important factors in deciding on the appropriateness is the issue of error. There are two basic errors for most of the applications in the quality world. They are (a) type alpha or type I error, the producer's error; it means that the producer is rejecting a good item and (b) type beta or type II error. This is the consumer's error. It means that the consumer is getting better quality than what he or she is paying for. *The way you as an organization (or management or team) define the error has a tremendous impact on how the sample is going to be defined and collected. Also, based on the definition of the error, the appropriate analysis will be selected, whether or not the analysis is proper and whether or not the experiment (study) was conducted based on sound design.*

7. Significance testing. One of the most troubling issues in quality today is the issue of significance. That is because both researchers and practitioners do not understand the concept fully. In everyday language the term *significance* means importance, whereas in statistics—this is very important—the term means probably true. The implication of these simple definitions is the fact that a particular study may be true without being important. As a result, when quality engineers say that a particular result is highly significant they mean that the result is very probably true. Under no circumstances do they mean that the result is highly important. Significance levels show you how probably true a result is. The most common level is 95 percent with no special significance, other than that the result has a 95 percent chance of being true. This is also misleading, however, due to the fact that most software packages show you .05, meaning that the finding has a 5 percent chance of not being true, which is the same as a 95 percent chance of being true. The 95 percent level comes from academic publications, where theory usually has to have at least a 95 percent chance of being true to be considered worth reporting. However, under no circumstances is the 95 percent level of significance sacred. It may be set at any level by the experimenter. In fact, in the business world, if something has a 90 percent chance of being true ($p = .1$), it certainly can't be considered proved, but it may be much better to act as if it were true rather than false.

To find the exact significance level, subtract the number shown from 1. For example, a value shown in the computer output as ".01" means there is a 99 percent ($1 - .01 = .99$) chance of being true. A strong warning about this significance is the fact that *it must be set a priori* before the experiment and analysis have taken place. Do not fall in the trap of seeing the significance on the computer printout and then changing the parameter of the significance.

STATISTICAL TOOLS

Once the preparation of the data is completed, we are ready to proceed with the analysis. There are many specific tools one can use in the analysis. Any statistics book can provide the reader with the mechanics of each of the tools. This section will discuss the two kinds of statistics and how to go about selecting the right one.

The two kinds of statistics are (1) descriptive and (2) inferential. Descriptive statistics are statistical methods concerned with describing or giving a clearer picture of the data. Typical examples are mean, median, standard deviation, Spearman rank correlation, and Pearson product-moment correlation, which are used to organize and summarize information about observations.

Inferential statistics are statistical methods concerned with inferring beyond the data. These methods attempt to draw conclusions about a population of things on the basis of observations of only a portion of the population. The experimenter uses a small sample of data, then draws inferences about the population, attempting to make reasonable decisions with incomplete information.

Inferential statistics are concerned with two types of problems:

1. An estimation of what the population is like. Estimation deals with ascertaining the magnitude of one or more universe parameters or the shape of the universe distribution.

2. Testing hypothesis about a population. Hypothesis testing is concerned with choosing among alternatives or establishing whether a specified parameter value or distribution shape is tenable based on sample evidence.

Note that the principles of estimation are needed in hypothesis testing. Hypothesis testing underlies, for example, the concept of a control chart, whereas establishing existing process capability is more of a problem of estimation.

Selection Process of Individual Statistical Tools

The number of choices available to the quality practitioner using either descriptive or inferential statistics is bountiful, and description of them all is beyond the scope of this chapter. However, because of the significance they offer we will summarize the process of selection of the most often used ones. The summary is shown in Figures 4–1 through Figure 4–3 and it is based on the three levels of data.

R E F E R E N C E S

Becker, W. E., and D. L. Harnett. *Business and Economics Statistics with Computer Applications.* Reading, Mass.: Addison-Wesley, 1987.

Deming, W. E. *Out of the Crisis.* Cambridge, Mass.: Massachusetts Institute of Technology, Center for Advanced Engineering Study, 1986.

———. *Some Theory of Sampling.* New York: Dover, 1966.

Freund, J. E., and F. J. Williams. *Elementary Statistics: The Modern Approach.* 2d ed. Englewood Cliffs, N.J.: Prentice Hall, 1972.

Hays, W. *Statistics.* New York: Holt, Rinehart & Winston, 1981.

Kerlinger, F. N. *Foundations of Behavioral Research.* 2d ed. New York: Holt, Rinehart & Winston, 1973.

Mansfield, E. *Statistics for Business and Economics: Methods and Applications.* 2d ed. New York: W. W. Norton, 1983.

Sharp, V. F. *Statistics for the Social Sciences.* Boston: Little, Brown, 1979.

CHAPTER 5

The Basic Tools of Quality

$\mathbf{A}$s in any endeavor, there are specific tools used to accomplish the defined tasks. Quality implementation is no different. In fact, the process and tools of implementing quality have become quite common. Much has been written in both areas (the process and the tools). The focus in this chapter is to offer a cursory systematic review of the basic tools and their application. To accomplish this task, I will address the 14-step training method, proceed with the applications of the tools, and then offer a short summary of each of the tools. For a detailed explanation and description, the reader is encouraged to see Montgomery (1985), Gitlow et al. (1989), Ishikawa (1982), Grant and Leavenworth (1980), *The Memory Jogger* (1988), and Gulezian (1991).

THE 14-STEP TRAINING METHOD

For the implementation process to be effective and timely, a systematic process must be in place. The process begins with the management recognizing some of the responsibilities of both training and the organization. Such recognition (perhaps through a needs assessment) will define the course of action both from a macro and micro perspective. The specific approach is delineated in the following 14 steps. I believe they are self-explanatory and offer no commentary.

The system (manager)—

1. Decides what is to be done.
2. Tells someone to do it.
3. Follows up to see if it has been done.
4. Discovers that it has not.
5. Asks why.
6. Finds out the employee didn't understand he (she) was supposed to do it.
7. Tells the employee again to do it.
8. Follows up once more to see if it has been done.
9. Discovers it has, but incorrectly.
10. Points out how it should have been done.
11. Follows up the next time to see if it has been done.
12. Discovers it has, but at the wrong time.
13. Points out when it should have been done.
14. Decides to do it himself (herself) next time.

The assumption of this training method is that a team is operating in the process and the manager is acting as a coach or director. For a complete discussion of the training model, see Stamatis (1995). Typical training approaches in healthcare are included in Appendix D.

APPLICATIONS FOR QUALITY IMPROVEMENT TOOLS

To know how to apply the basic tools for quality improvement, we must first understand the steps of problem solving. To be sure, there is no specific number of steps. However, *all* problem solving approaches have some basic criteria as their core approach. Some have defined it as the scientific method: (1) set a hypothesis, (2) test the hypothesis, (3) analyze results, and (4) reject or accept the hypothesis. Others have defined it as an eight-step approach (Stamatis 1995; Ford 1987).

To demonstrate that a problem-solving approach is not unique, I offer a variation for healthcare in Table 5–1. It is based on four basic steps, but each step has several substeps. The overall ap-

T A B L E   5–1

Problem-Solving Approach

Category	Basic Steps	Tools Used
Define problem	1. List and prioritize problem(s)	Data collection
	2. Define project and team	Process flow diagram
Research problem	1. Analyze symptoms	Flow diagrams, data collection, Pareto analysis, brainstorming
	2. Set hypothesis	Brainstorming, cause-and-effect diagram
	3. Test hypothesis	Brainstorming, data collection, graphs, flow diagrams, Pareto analysis, scatter diagrams, control charts
	4. Get to the root cause	Data collection, flow diagrams, graphs, Pareto analysis, scatter diagrams, control charts
Fix problem	1. Find alternative solutions	Brainstorming, cause-and-effect diagram, flow diagram
	2. Define solutions and controls	Data collection, flow diagram, graphs, scatter diagrams, control charts
	3. Plan for resistance to change	Brainstorming
	4. Implement solutions and controls	Flow diagrams
Monitor process	1. Monitor performance	Data collection, graphs and charts, Pareto analysis, histograms, control charts
	2. Monitor control system	Data collection, graphs and charts, control charts

proach involves 12 individual steps. In no way is this approach better or worse than any other; it is simply different.

SUMMARY OF THE BASIC TOOLS

As mentioned earlier, it is beyond the scope of this book to address in detail the basic tools of quality. However, because of their importance to the whole improvement process, their frequent use, and their simplicity, each is summarized.

Brainstorming

Brainstorming is a group decision-making technique designed to generate a large number of creative ideas through an interactive process. It encourages creative thinking to generate alternative ideas to be considered in making decisions. The basis for such creativity is synergy, which is defined as the whole is greater than the sum of its parts. The team can use brainstorming to get its ideas organized into a process flow diagram or a cause-and-effect diagram.

Questions That Can Be Used during Brainstorming Sessions

Often the question regarding brainstorming is, How do we begin? The following five questions pose a good beginning:

1. What are the organization's three most important unsolved and/or recurrent quality problems as you see them?
2. What kind of action plan is needed to solve these problems?
3. Which areas are most in need of such action? (Try to be as specific as possible.)
4. What are some major obstacles in the way of improving quality?
5. Must we follow rules if it is a creative session? Yes. Specific rules are necessary, and they are:
   a. Clearly define the goal of the brainstorming session. This is very important. If the definition is not clear, the participants will be discussing different problems.
   b. Try to have *all* participants give their ideas in three words or less.
   c. Write down *all* ideas. Some may seem silly but they may lead to an idea that could help solve the problem. Generate a large number of ideas. Quantity, not quality, is important here. The greater the idea count, the better! Combinations of ideas are OK, too.
   d. Do not allow one or two individuals to dominate the session.

  e. Make the ideas visible so that everyone can easily see
  them. If you have an overhead projector, you can list
  the ideas on a transparency. Or use a flip chart.

Brainstorming Procedures

In addition to the rules, there are appropriate procedures that must
be followed for an optimum resolution. These procedures are divided into two categories: creating ideas and evaluating ideas.

Creating Ideas

  1. The leader asks each person to list ideas on a piece of
paper.
  2. The leader then solicits everyone's contribution. This is
done by going from person to person in rotation. If a member does
not have an idea on a particular round, that person simply says, "I
pass." However, each participant is called on at every round.
  3. As ideas are given, someone should list them on a transparency or a flip chart.
  4. Omit *only* ideas you already have listed.
  5. After all participants have contributed their individual
lists, the leader asks for any additional ideas that may have been
generated during the contribution process.
  6. The human mind thinks at two different levels, the conscious and the unconscious. After a good brainstorming session
everyone's mind will be spinning with new, wild ideas. The unconscious mind will continue brainstorming even after you've
stopped thinking about it at a conscious level. Thus, the team
should continue the brainstorming session after an incubation period has passed.

Evaluating the Ideas

  1. Evaluate each idea. Some ideas will be scrapped right
away without a detailed discussion.
  2. Direct the evaluation toward the idea and *never* toward the
person who suggested it.

Process Flow Diagram

One of the most used and powerful tools in the quality improvement process is a process flow diagram, which is a road map of the
process (Figure 5–1). Specifically, a process flow diagram illus-

FIGURE 5-1

Streamlined Retro Bill Process Flow Diagram

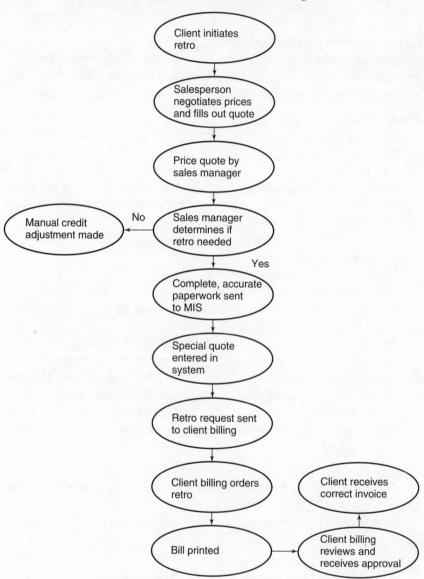

trates and clarifies events/tasks in a process and the events/tasks between them. This diagram assists in highlighting the present situation, differences between what should or is thought to be happening and the actual situation, the proposed situation, and potential problem areas. A process flow diagram can be used to facilitate effectiveness during brainstorming, cause and effect diagram construction, and in every other situation where there is an ambivalence about what the present state is. To construct a process flow diagram, the following are important:

Steps for Constructing a Process Flow Diagram

1. Assemble *all* appropriate people.
2. Define the process and its boundaries.
3. Brainstorm the process.
4. Use the simplest symbols possible, that is, ○ for operations, D for delay, → for flow, inverted delta for inventory, and square for inspection; decisions are usually shown as diamonds or circles since they are activities (operations).*
5. Draw the steps the process actually follows.
6. Make sure each feedback loop is accounted for.
7. Draw the steps the process should follow.
8. Compare the two, and make the appropriate adjustments.

Check Sheet

Check sheets are forms that guide the experimenter in categorizing the data as they are being collected (Figure 5–2). Its construction is simple.

Steps for Constructing a Check Sheet

1. Agree on the item being observed.
2. Decide on time period to collect data.

---

* □ or ○ = Operation
D = Delay
→ = Flow
∇ = Inventory
□ = Inspection
◇ = Decisions

FIGURE 5–2

Sample Check Sheet

Reason	Monday	Tuesday	Wednesday	Thursday	Friday	**Total**
Money	|||||	||	|	|||||	||||| ||	20
Sex	||	||	||	||	||	10
Children	|||||	||	||||| ||	|	||||	19
Total	12	6	10	8	13	49

3. Design a form that is clear and easy to understand.
4. Collect the data honestly and consistently.

Histogram

A histogram is a bar graph that gives a historical and at the same time a pictorial representation of a set of data (Figure 5–3). It is used to determine the:

- Shape of a series of data values.
- Readiness of a process to undergo a capability study.
- Dispersion and central tendency of the data (quick analysis).
- Relationship of machines, customers, suppliers, and so on (quick analysis).

Steps for Constructing a Histogram

1. Determine how many data values to use.
2. Determine the width of the data by computing the range.
3. Select the number of cells for the histogram.

F I G U R E   5–3

Sample Histogram of the Height of Men

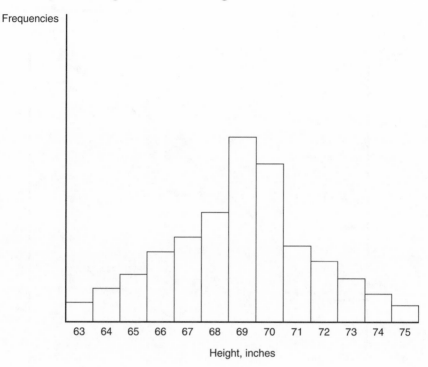

Height, inches

4. Determine the width of each cell.
5. Determine the starting number for the first interval.
6. Calculate the intervals.
7. Assign data values to the appropriate intervals.
8. Construct the histogram by drawing bars to represent the cell frequencies.

Pareto Chart

The Pareto analysis is a chart based on the Pareto principle (Figure 5–4). This principle was named for an Italian economist who in the late 1800s found that most of the wealth in Italy was owned by a few of the people. Today we find—as an extension of this princi-

FIGURE 5-4

Pareto Chart on Customer Complaints

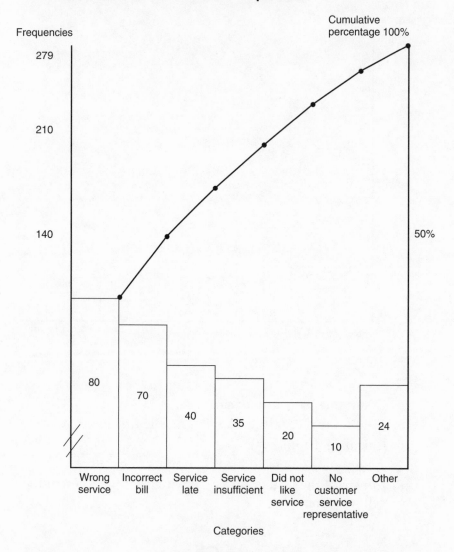

ple—that 80 percent of our problems in the hospital or the office can be traced to 20 percent of the causes. The Pareto analysis is a process of ranking opportunities so we can determine which should be pursued first. In essence, the Pareto analysis allows us to separate for examination the vital few from the trivial many.

Pareto analysis should be used at various stages in a quality improvement program to determine which step to take next. Pareto analysis is used to answer questions such as "Which department should have the next team?" or "On what problem should we concentrate our efforts?"

To construct a Pareto chart, the following steps are necessary.

Steps for Constructing a Pareto Chart

1. Decide the appropriate time interval.
2. Decide the number of classifications.
3. Decide the total number of occurrences for each category using primary or secondary data.
4. Calculate the category percentage.
5. Rank categories in descending order.
6. Calculate the cumulative percentage.
7. Construct a Pareto chart for magnitudes and cumulative percentages.

The chart itself is a graph that ranks factors in descending order of frequency or magnitude from left to right, in the following manner:

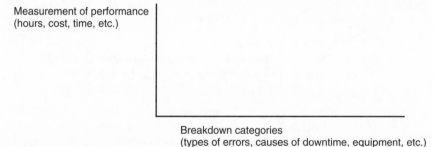

Measurement of performance
(hours, cost, time, etc.)

Breakdown categories
(types of errors, causes of downtime, equipment, etc.)

Cause-and-Effect Diagram

A cause-and-effect diagram, also called a fishbone diagram and the Ishikawa diagram, is a method of organizing information about a problem or a goal (Figure 5–5). It is a visual representation of what people think are the causes of a particular problem. In its simplest form it is a method used to help decide what to do to achieve a goal, based on the relationship among the variables of "5Ms & E": manpower (people), machine, method, material, measurement, and environment. With the analysis of the relationships between these variables, an isolated cause-and-effect resolution is identified.

There are three basic rules in constructing this diagram:

Steps for Constructing a Cause-and-Effect Diagram

1. Start with a clear definition of the problem or goal. Put this in a box on the right side of the paper.

2. Draw arrows using the "5Ms & E": manpower, machine, method, material, measurement, and environment. Other labels may be used if appropriate and applicable.

3. Begin to fill in all the things that you think will cause the problem or help achieve the goal.

A typical cause-and-effect diagram appears in Figure 5–5a. Because this diagram is very popular in the quality improvement process, let us address some issues in the construction process.

1. A cause-and-effect diagram may be constructed at the same time that the brainstorming is being conducted, after a process flow diagram is completed, or even independently from either one of them.

2. Write down in the applicable category everything people suggest; do not judge.

3. Remember, the information is important, *not* the form.

4. Where causes are put in the diagram is not important at first; they can go under any of the headings or even multiple headings.

5. There is nothing wrong with placing the same cause in different places on the diagram if people want it that way (if you find that a cause is recurring under different headings, it may be an indication of obvious trouble).

6. It is important for all persons to help in adding causes to the diagram.

7. If the diagram is not finished at the end of the meeting, you or others can add to it later.

8. Some companies post cause-and-effect diagrams so that their employees can add to them; they serve as displays rather than tools to identify problems and improvements.

F I G U R E   5–5

Cause-and-Effect Diagram Skeleton and Example of a Cause-and-Effect Diagram: Retro Bill

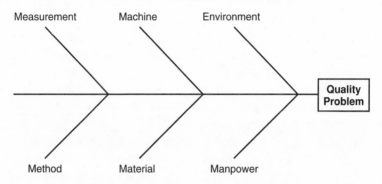

a.

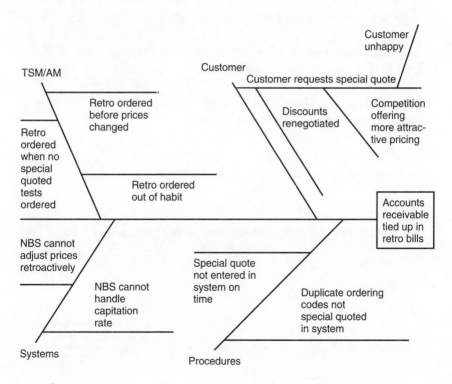

b.

Dispersion Analysis
Cause-and-Effect Diagram

A major disadvantage of the cause-and-effect diagram is that many major causes for a quality problem could appear on a single branch. This makes the diagram difficult to develop and use. A slightly different cause-and-effect diagram is a dispersion analysis diagram in which all the major sources of variability are listed as branches (Figure 5–6). Often the cause-and-effect diagram is used first, and then the dispersion analysis diagram is used to identify and expand on the major causes.

In choosing the cause-and-effect type of diagram versus other types, consider its advantages and disadvantages. Its advantages are a clear grouping of potential causes that enables effective later analysis and a resulting diagram that is not too complex. Its disadvantages are that major causes can be easily overlooked, if the 5Ms & E method is not used first; it is sometimes difficult to classify major causes; and greater knowledge of potential causes is required.

In construction of this diagram, the question is, Why is there variability in major cause (#) that could cause quality problem (X)?

How to Use a Dispersion Analysis
Cause-and-Effect Diagram

There are many ways that the dispersion analysis diagram may be used. However, for an effective and efficient use in the workplace, the following seven rules should be followed:

F I G U R E   5–6

Dispersion Analysis Cause-and-Effect Diagram

1. Develop a process flow diagram for the part of the process you want to improve.
2. Isolate and clearly define the problem to be solved.
3. Use the brainstorming technique to find all possible causes of the quality problem.
4. Organize the brainstorming results into logical categories.
5. Construct the appropriate cause-and-effect diagram that clearly and accurately displays the relationship of all the data in each category.
6. Explore and implement solutions to assess improvement.
7. Use statistical methods to assess improvement.

Selecting a Dispersion Analysis Diagram

Because a dispersion analysis diagram is used to identify and categorize problems, the person who is using it must be cognizant of some basic information as far as selecting a solution is concerned. The information is gained through a series of questions. The following questions may serve as samples.

- Will the solution solve our problem, and is there information existing to improve this?
- How long is it going to take to make the necessary changes and to see some signs of reducing or eliminating the problem?
- What monetary investment will be needed?
- What quality improvements will be achieved?
- How many people and jobs are affected by the quality improvement solution?
- How will the improvement affect people? Will they need to make changes? Will they choose to accept the changes?
- What technical changes are needed? Will these changes have an impact on the 5Ms & E?
- How much change can the company absorb at one time? How quickly can the changes be made and who is needed to help make the changes?

In addition to these questions, the team must use some rules for selecting a solution and then move to the approval process. The rules are very basic but very important in the process. They provide consistency as well as a systematic approach to the dispersion analysis cause-and-effect process. On the other hand, the approval process provides a sort of checklist of how the solution is approved and then implemented. To monitor the process, an action plan is used (see Figures 1–4, 1–5, and 1–6 for the appropriate form). The rules, approval process, and implementation steps are as follows:

Rules for Selecting a Solution

1. Decide your goal (what you want to accomplish) and the method you are going to use to solve the problem.
2. Be sure to let all the people who are affected by the problem be involved in selecting and planning its solution.
3. Evaluate the costs, benefits, and time involved to implement the solution.
4. Decide the steps that are necessary to implement the solution.
5. Create a formal presentation for choosing the problem and your suggested solution or solutions.

Approval Process

1. Introduction: Tell them what you are going to talk about.
2. Clearly define the problem.
3. Show the importance of the problem and its related costs (use evidence).
4. Clearly state your proposed solution.
5. Talk about the benefits of solving this problem (use evidence).
6. State what is needed to solve the problem.
7. Prepare a checklist to cover anticipated questions and objections.

Implementing the Solution

1. Clarify all tasks to be completed.
2. Define the order of completion of the tasks.
3. What are the resources needed to complete each task. Who does what? How long will it take?
4. Determine the time frame for completion of the task.

5. Assign responsibility for each task.

6. Assign how results will be measured and monitored.

7. Set up procedures for measuring results of each task.

8. Evaluate effectiveness of the solution.

The team has responsibilities for effective implementation of a solution. They are:

- Do not take anything for granted.
- Do not assume—ask questions.
- Each person needs to know what they are responsible for doing.
- Everyone works to complete and follow through with the action plan.
- Make sure completion of assignments is monitored.
- Remove any barriers to successfully implementing the solution.
- Be sure everyone affected by the solution is in the final process of implementation.

Scatter Plot

If one is interested in finding out if there is a relationship between variables, the scatter plot is a useful tool for finding that relationship (Figure 5–7). Regardless of what the relationship is or shows, the scatter plot *under no circumstances* can prove that one variable *causes* the other. What it shows in a graphical form is that a relationship exists and how strong that relationship is.

One of the shortcomings of the scatter plot is that it is not always possible to describe a relationship with a mathematical formula (it is a pictorial relationship). In statistics it is possible to numerically describe the relationship between two sets of data. The methods used to do this are too difficult to present here, but we can gain an idea of the result of the methods. A relationship between sets of data is called a correlation.

Steps in Constructing a Scatter Plot

1. Collect at least 50 paired samples of data.

2. Draw horizontal and vertical axes, making sure that the

F I G U R E   5–7

Scatter Plots

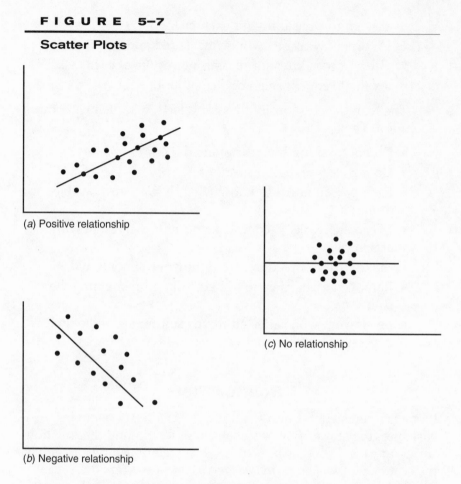

(a) Positive relationship

(c) No relationship

(b) Negative relationship

values on each axis become higher as you move away from the origin (as you move up and to the right in the vertical and horizontal axes respectively.) As a general rule, the expected cause is the horizontal axis, and the effect is the vertical axis.

3. Plot the data. A typical plotting is shown in Figure 5–7.

STATISTICAL PROCESS CONTROL

Statistical process control (SPC) is a bundle of techniques that identify random (common cause) versus identifiable (special) causes in a process. Both of these are potential sources for improvement. The amount of random variation effects the capability of a machine to produce within a desired range of dimensions.

Hence, SPC could be performed to determine processing capabilities and how to achieve those levels. The determination and correction of recurring systematic changes is also a possibility.

The reduction of the random variation or the uncertainty of a process and the identification and correction of special causes are critical aspects of the total quality management process. Correction often requires a change in the total process and quite often multiple changes at the same time.

The first step of process improvement is to control the environment and the components of the system so that variations are within natural predictable limits. The second step is to reduce the underlying variation of the process. The undertaking of both of these represents the issue of control charting.

Control Chart

A control chart is a pictorial representation of the process variation over time. A control chart identifies the changes in the process and, unless the characteristic of the process is known, the change cannot be determined. All control charts are fundamentally based on the normal distribution with statistical limits. The limits (upper and lower) are calculated and are drawn on either side of the process average. Do not confuse limits with specifications. Limits are calculated based on data from the process. Specifications are given by the customer and are the requirements we are expected to meet as a very minimum. See Figure 5–8 for the relationship between control limits and specifications.

In a sense, a control chart is a tool that sends a signal, making possible the distinction between abnormal and normal variation. In addition, one of the fundamental concepts in all control charts is the notion of control. Control *does not* necessarily mean that the product or service will meet your needs. It means only that the process is consistent and, even then, it may be consistently bad or good. For a detailed discussion on control theory and application, see Montgomery (1985) and Duncan (1986).

Types of Control Charts

There are many types of control charts. However, their selection depends on the kind of data available. See Figure 5–9 for a guide for selection. As already discussed, there are two kinds of data: (1)

F I G U R E   5–8

Relationship between Control Limits and Specifications

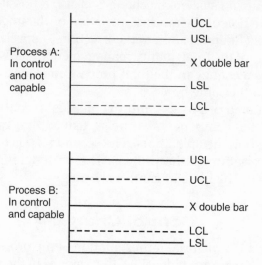

UCL = Upper control limit, process dependent

LCL = Lower control limit, process dependent

LSL = Lower specification, limit customer dependent

USL = Upper specification limit, customer dependent

X double bar = Overall average

variable and (2) attribute. When variable data are available, there is great flexibility to use some of the most powerful charts available. Variable control charts monitor or measure things that are actually measurable on a continuous scale such as temperature, pressure, acidity, time, and so forth. For example, typical charts that may be used in monitoring variable data are:

X-bar and R chart   This chart requires a number of consecutive units be taken n times per work period and analyzed for specific criteria. It graphically displays process stability and shows data in terms of spread (piece-to-piece variability) and location (process average). The X-bar covers averages of values in small subgroups (sample taken), known as measure of location. The R

F I G U R E   5–9

A Guide for Choosing Selected Control Charts

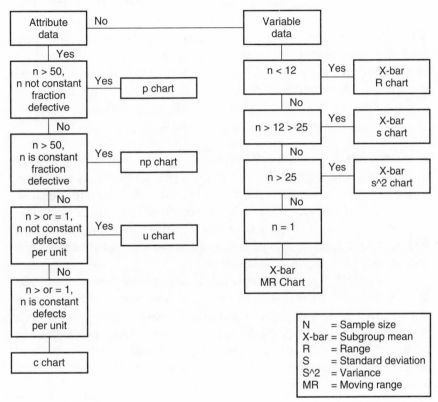

chart deals with the range of values within each sample (highest minus lowest), known as measure of spread.

Individual and moving range chart   This standard control chart requires fewer samples than the X-bar and R chart to establish stability. Even with one sample, a person can use this chart to establish trends and identify the variation between batches and/or individual items. Other than the level of sampling, this chart is very similar to the X-bar and R chart.

Median and R chart   This is a standard chart that is an alternative to the X-bar and R chart for the control of processes. It is less sensitive to trends, however, and under some circumstances is considered to be more difficult to construct. It graphically displays the stability of a process. The chart yields similar information to the X bar and R chart but has several advantages: (1) It is easier to use; daily calculations are not required. (2) Individual values and medians are plotted, and the median chart shows spread of process output and gives an ongoing view of process variation. (3) It shows where nonconformities are scattered through a more or less continuous flow of a function. (4) It shows where nonconformities from different areas may be evident.

X-bar and s chart   This is a standard control chart similar to the X-bar and R chart, however, the s part of the chart considers standard deviation and is more complicated to calculate. Because of the standard deviation, it is more sensitive to the process variation, especially with larger samples. On the other hand, it is less sensitive in detecting special causes of variation that produce only one value in a subgroup as unusual.

Conversely, attribute control charts result from counting. They monitor or measure whether variables do or do not have certain characteristics or how often characteristics are present in a process. Examples are: delays, percentage of defects, percentage of nonconformities. Basically, these control charts monitor pass/fail or go/no go situations. When the data are attribute in nature, then we should use different charts. For example:

p-chart   This is a standard control chart requiring a constant sample size. It charts either conforming or nonconforming items. Graphically, it displays stability of the process. The p-chart measures actual number of conforming and nonconforming items rather than total number of faults. It expresses numbers in either fractional or percentile terms (whether conforming or nonconforming items are used) of the total sample, for example, total number of faulty forms in a batch irrespective of the number of faults in any one form.

np-chart   This standard control chart is similar to the c-chart, but must be used if the sample sizes vary. Graphically, it displays stability of the process. It measures number of nonconforming items rather than total number of faults, for example, total number of faulty forms in a batch irrespective of the faults in any one form.

c-chart   This standard control chart is for the total number of nonconformities based on a constant sample size. Graphically, this chart displays stability of the process, for example, total number of errors in a batch of 100 forms rather than just the number of faulty forms.

u-chart   Standard control chart that is similar to the c-chart, but must be used if the sample sizes vary. Graphically, it displays stability of the process, for example, total number of errors in a batch of 100 forms rather than just the number of faulty forms.

The steps for constructing each of these charts are given below.

Steps for Constructing an X-bar and R Chart

1. Select the size, frequency, and number of subgroups.

2. Select and record raw data.

3. Calculate the average and range of each of the subgroups.

4. Calculate the overall average of the process as well as the average range.

5. Construct the control chart scale. (A good rule of thumb to follow in constructing the scale is the following: For the range chart, you take two to three times the largest range average. For the average chart, you identify the largest and the smallest average of each of the subgroups, then take the difference of these two. Then you multiply the difference by 2 and add it to the grand average.)

6. Plot averages and ranges on the chart.

7. Calculate control limits for the range chart, using appropriate formulas and constants (see Appendix F, Part II).

8. Calculate control limits for the average chart, using appropriate formulas and constants.

9. Interpret the range chart.

10. Interpret the average chart.

If the process is consistent and repeatable then,

11. Calculate the process capability.

12. Continue to monitor the process.

If the process is not consistent and repeatable then,

   11. Identify the cause or causes of inconsistency.

   12. Remove the cause(s).

   13. Continue to monitor until the process becomes consistent and repeatable.

   14. Move to step 11.

Steps for Constructing an Average and Standard Deviation (SD) Chart

   1. Select the size, frequency, and number of subgroups.

   2. Select and record raw data.

   3. Calculate the average, range, and SD of each of the subgroups.

   4. Calculate the overall average of the process, the average range, and the average SD of the process.

   5. Construct the control chart scale. (A good rule of thumb to follow in constructing the scale is the following: For the SD chart, you take two to three times the largest SD average. For the average chart, you identify the largest and the smallest average of each of the subgroups, then take the difference of these two. Then you multiply the difference by 2 and add it to the grand average.)

   6. Plot averages and ranges on the chart.

   7. Calculate control limits for the SD chart, using appropriate formulas and constants.

   8. Calculate control limits for the average chart, using appropriate formulas and constants.

   9. Interpret the SD chart.

   10. Interpret the average chart.

If the process is consistent and repeatable then,

   11. Calculate the process capability.

   12. Continue to monitor the process.

If the process is not consistent and repeatable then,

   11. Identify the cause or causes of inconsistency.

   12. Remove the cause(s).

   13. Continue to monitor until the process becomes consistent and repeatable.

   14. Move to step 11.

Steps for Constructing an Individual and Moving Range Chart

   1. Collect and record raw data.

   2. Select the appropriate interval of samples.

3. Calculate the range of each of the interval subgroups.

4. Calculate the overall average of the process as well as the average range.

5. Construct the control chart scale.

6. Plot averages and ranges on the chart. (A good rule of thumb to follow in constructing the scale is the following: For the range chart, you take two to three times the largest range average. For the individual chart, you identify the largest and the smallest value, then take the difference of these two. Then you multiply the difference by 2 and add it to the grand average.)

7. Calculate control limits for the range chart, using appropriate formulas and constants.

8. Calculate control limits for the average chart, using appropriate formulas and constants.

9. Interpret the range chart.

10. Interpret the average chart.

If the process is consistent and repeatable then,

11. Calculate the process capability.

12. Continue to monitor the process.

If the process is not consistent and repeatable then,

11. Identify the cause or causes of inconsistency.

12. Remove the cause(s).

13. Continue to monitor until the process becomes consistent and repeatable.

14. Move to step 11.

Steps for Constructing the Median and Range Chart

1. Select the size, frequency, and number of subgroups.

2. Select and record raw data.

3. Select the median of each of the subgroups as well as the range.

4. Select the overall median of the process as well as the average range.

5. Construct the control chart scale. (A good rule of thumb to follow in constructing the scale is the following: For the range chart, you take two to three times the largest range average. For the median chart, you identify the largest and the smallest median of each of the subgroups, then take the difference of these two. Then you multiply the difference by 2 and add it to the grand median.)

6. Plot median values and ranges on the chart.

7. Calculate control limits for the range chart, using appropriate formulas and constants.

8. Calculate control limits for the median chart, using appropriate formulas and constants.

9. Interpret the range chart.

10. Interpret the median chart.

If the process is consistent and repeatable then,

11. Calculate the process capability.

12. Continue to monitor the process.

If the process is not consistent and repeatable then,

11. Identify the cause or causes of inconsistency.

12. Remove the cause(s).

13. Continue to monitor until the process becomes consistent and repeatable.

14. Move to step 11.

Steps for Constructing a p-chart

1. Select the size, frequency, and number of subgroups.

2. Collect and record raw data.

3. Calculate the proportion for each subgroup.

4. Calculate the average proportion as well as the average number of defectives.

5. Construct the control chart scale. (A good rule of thumb to follow in constructing the scale is the following: For the p-chart, you identify the largest and the smallest proportion of each of the subgroups, then take the difference of these two. Then you multiply the difference by 2 and add it to the grand average.)

6. Plot individual proportions.

7. Calculate control limits using appropriate formulas.

9. Interpret the p-chart.

If the process is consistent and repeatable then,

10. Calculate the process capability.

11. Continue to monitor the process.

If the process is not consistent and repeatable then,

10. Identify the cause or causes of inconsistency.

11. Remove the cause(s).

12. Continue to monitor and watch for process change.

13. Move to step 10.

Steps for Constructing an np-Chart
1. Select the size, frequency, and number of subgroups.
2. Collect and record raw data.
3. Calculate the process average number of nonconformities.
4. Construct control chart scale. (A good rule of thumb to follow in constructing the scale is the following: For the np-chart, you identify the largest and the smallest proportion of each of the subgroups, then take the difference of these two. Then you multiply the difference by 2 and add it to the grand proportion.)
5. Calculate control limits based on appropriate formulas.
6. Interpret the control chart.
If the process is consistent then,
7. Calculate the process capability.
If the process is not consistent then,
7. Identify and remove inconsistencies.
8. Continue to monitor and watch for changes in the process.

Steps for Constructing a c-Chart
1. Select the size, frequency, and number of subgroups.
2. Collect and record raw data.
3. Calculate the process average number of nonconformities.
4. Construct the control chart scale. (A good rule of thumb to follow in constructing the scale is the following: For the c-chart, you identify the largest and the smallest defectives of each of the subgroups, then take the difference of these two. Then you multiply the difference by 2 and add it to the grand average defective.)
5. Calculate control limits based on appropriate formulas.
6. Interpret the control chart.
If the process is consistent then,
7. Calculate the process capability.
If the process is not consistent then,
7. Identify and remove inconsistencies.
8. Continue to monitor and watch for changes in the process.

Steps for Constructing a u-Chart
1. Select the size, frequency, and number of subgroups.
2. Collect and record raw data.
3. Record and plot the nonconformities per unit in each subgroup.

4. Calculate the process average number of nonconformities per unit.

5. Construct the control chart scale. (A good rule of thumb to follow in constructing the scale is the following: For the u-chart, you identify the largest and the smallest nonconformities of each of the subgroups, then take the difference of these two. Then you multiply the difference by 2 and add it to the grand average nonconformities.)

6. Calculate control limits based on appropriate formulas.

7. Interpret the control chart.

If the process is consistent then,

8. Calculate the process capability.

If the process is not consistent then,

7. Identify and remove inconsistencies.

8. Continue to monitor and watch for changes in the process.

REFERENCES

Duncan, A. J. *Quality Control and Industrial Statistics.* 5th ed. Homewood, Ill.: Irwin, 1986.

Gitlow, H.; S. Gitlow; A. Oppenheim; and R. Oppenheim. *Tools and Methods for the Improvement of Quality.* Homewood, Ill.: Irwin, 1989.

Grant, E. L., and R. S. Leavenworth. *Statistical Quality Control.* 5th ed. New York: McGraw- Hill, 1980.

Gulezian, R. *Process Control Statistical Principles and Tools.* New York: Quality Alert Institute, 1991.

Ishikawa K. *Guide to Quality Control.* White Plains, N.Y.: Kraus International Publications (Asian Productivity Organization), 1982.

The Memory Jogger. Methuen, Mass.: GOAL/QPC, 1988.

Montgomery, D. C. *Introduction to Statistical Quality Control.* New York: John Wiley & Sons, 1985.

Stamatis, D. H. *Total Quality Service.* Delray Beach, Fla.: St. Lucie Press, 1995.

Team Oriented Problem Solving. Dearborn, Mich.: Ford Motor Co. Power Train Operations, 1987.

CHAPTER 6

Other Common Quality Tools Used in Healthcare

When solving a quality problem, it is critical to attack the underlying cause of the problem and not the symptoms. The underlying cause can be identified by listing all possible causes and identifying the most probable cause based on the definition of the problem and data collection, followed by the appropriate and applicable analysis. This analysis requires specific tools. In the field of quality, besides the basic tools addressed in the last chapter, there are other tools and charts that the quality professional may use when appropriate. This chapter focuses on several of the most often used tools in the pursuit of quality. By no means are these the only ones. It is beyond the scope of this book to address all of them. However, the reader is highly encouraged to see additional references in which the tools and charts can be found, for example, Shigeru (1988), Burr (1989), *Improvement Tools* (1991), Delbecq and Van de Ven (1986), Duncan (1986), Brassard (1989), Stamatis (1995), Montgomery (1985), Gitlow et al. (1989), Ishikawa (1982), Grant and Leavenworth (1980), *The Memory Jogger* (1988), and Gulezian (1991).

INTERNAL ASSESSMENT SURVEYS

An internal assessment of strengths and weaknesses can be used to identify quality improvement projects. This can take the form of "gap analysis," "needs assessment," or "surveys," and so on.

Whatever the selection process, the final determination can be made using a team approach and sound business strategy. The specific determination process may be followed by team discussion or by using the nominal group process (discussed in this chapter). The assessment—however it is conducted—can be made by the owner of a product, process, or service and/or by the department being served. An internal assessment can also be approached from the viewpoint of the generic value-added chain. For each block of the chain, two questions can be asked:

What are the alternatives for least cost operation?

What are the alternatives to provide differentiation?

The value-added chain can also provide customer perspective by suggesting these questions:

How does our product or service help customers minimize their cost?

How does our product or service help customers to differentiate their product or service?

RUN (TREND) CHARTING

Historical data can be used to develop statistical forecasts and confidence intervals that depict acceptable random variation. See Figure 6–1 for an example of a run chart. When data fall within the confidence intervals, there is no cause to suspect unusual behavior (variation). However, data outside of the confidence intervals could provide an opportunity for improvement. It might also be informative to pursue improvement as a device to reduce the range of variation or the size of the confidence interval.

FORCE FIELD ANALYSIS

Force field analysis (FFA) is a systematic way of identifying and portraying the forces (quite often people) for or against change in an organization. The specific forces will be different depending on the area where they are applied. Typical steps in conducting an FFA are:

F I G U R E   6–1

Run Chart
Autochemistry Reagent Consumption

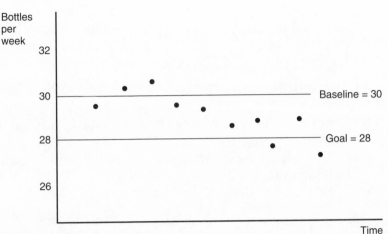

1. Define the current situation.
2. Define the desired position based on the results of an FFA.
3. Define the worst possible situation.
4. What are the forces for change, and what is their relative strength?
5. What are the forces against change, and what is their relative strength?
6. What forces can you influence?
7. Define the specific action to be taken relative to each of these forces that you can influence.

NOMINAL GROUP PROCESS

This technique was developed by A. L. Delbecq and A. H. Van de Ven (1986) and is a structured group process used to help make decisions. One of the greatest advantages of this method is that all members of the team can participate and have an equal voice. It is used when one needs to generate and choose a course of action for improvement. It is a priority setting tool for decision making. The nominal group process is composed of the following six steps:

1. Identify and define the area of opportunity.
2. Silently generate action items on how to improve. Each member independently writes down action items, using as few words as possible or short phrases.
3. State and record the ideas that each member has identified.
4. Discuss each item on the list.
5. Establish criteria for voting. The criteria must be easy to implement and must be effective.
6. Conduct a preliminary vote based on forced ranking. The steps are:
   a. Individuals choose the items most important to them.
   b. Rank order the outcome.
   c. Record the votes.
   d. Discuss the results of the vote.

THE FIVE WHYS

When identifying underlying causes, it can also be useful to ask five sequential "whys" to get to the heart of a problem. For example, if the problem is that microbiology specimens are not fully incubated by 8 AM, ask:

Why does this happen? Specimens sit on trays outside hoods for long periods.

Why? Technicians are not working at the hood when specimens arrive.

Why? Technicians are doing ova and parasite testing.

Why? Ova and parasite tests are always done first.

Why? Current work flow prioritization puts ova and parasite testing ahead of specimen incubation.

AFFINITY CHART

An affinity chart is the organized output from a team brainstorming session. It differs from brainstorming, in that it uses cards as headers that can be changed and organized in piles for discussion. The affinity chart was created by Kawakita Jiro and is also known as the KJ method. The purpose of an affinity chart is to generate, organize, and consolidate information concerning a product, process, service and/or complex issue or problem. The chart is used when the answer to the following three questions is yes.

Is the issue complex and hard to understand?

Is the problem uncertain, disorganized, or overwhelming?

Does the problem require the involvement and support of a group or a team?

The actual construction of the chart takes seven basic steps:

1. Choose a group leader.
2. Choose the problem and, if possible, state it in a question form.
3. Brainstorm and record *all* ideas; each idea should be written on its own index card or adhesive note.
4. Arrange the cards into like categories.
5. Name each category with a header card.
6. Draw the affinity chart; arrange headers with the appropriate generated ideas and circle or box them together.
7. Discuss the categories.

RELATIONS DIAGRAM

A relations diagram is a pictorial representation of the cause-and-effect relationships among the elements of a problem or issue (Figure 6–2). The purpose of this diagram is to identify the root causes and effects of a problem. It is used when the answer to the following two questions is yes.

Do the aspects of a complex issue need to be analyzed and understood?

Is the team having trouble getting to the root causes of a problem because only symptoms seem to be apparent?

The steps for generating the diagram are as follows:

1. Identify a clear definition of the problem.
2. Construct the diagram layout. The problem statement is put in the center of a sheet of paper with the header cards all around it.

F I G U R E   6–2

A Relations Diagram

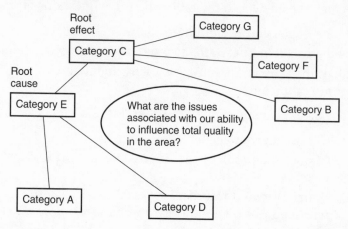

3. Analyze the relationships. Analyze each header with the other header cards, always asking the question, Does this category influence others, or is it influenced by the others? A line is drawn between the categories if there is a relationship, and an arrow points to that relationship.

4. Count the arrows.

5. Identify the root causes and effects. The root causes are the categories with the greatest number of arrows going out. The root effects are the categories with the greatest number of arrows going in.

6. Study the final diagram. Make the decision.

STORYTELLING

Quality improvement storyboards and storybooks use the steps in the FOCUS-PDCA strategy to help teams organize their work and their presentations so others can more readily learn from them. They reduce variation in the process by focusing the learning experience on the content rather than the method of telling. A typical structure for storytelling is shown in Figure 6–3. In addition, storybooks form a permanent record of a team's actions and achievements and all the data generated. Storyboards also can function as the working minutes of the team.

FIGURE   6-3

Example of a Storyboard Skeleton

F	C	
O	U	
S		
Team road map		

DECISION MATRIX

A decision matrix is a variation of the nominal group process. It may be used with complex problems. A decision matrix is a sheet made up of columns and rows. The sheet displays the following information.

1. Write possible improvement actions down the left column.
2. Write the criteria across the top of the sheet.
3. Weigh each criterion.
4. Rate each idea.
5. Multiply the ratings and weighting factors.
6. Add the weighted ratings.

PROGRAM EVALUATION REVIEW TECHNIQUE

The Program Evaluation Review Technique (PERT) is a tool used by project managers to identify certain elements about the project, such as critical path, early finish time, late finish time, and slack time. The PERT approach is to identify the critical path of the project and plan in such a way that no bottlenecks or other difficulties will be likely to occur in the implementation process of the specific project. To make sure this occurs, the PERT analysis involves a project network structure.

A network is, in essence, a "hooking" together of many activities that make up a project. For example, a timetable or a budget or a delivery may represent the project structure. However, these activities may be thought of as crude devices, since they imply that each activity starts only after the previous one is completed. To further clarify this point, let us examine a timetable structure. Strictly speaking, the timetable obscures the possibility of carrying on some activities simultaneously to reach an earlier project completion date.

Activity is the key concept in PERT. An activity is any action involving the use of resources and occurring over time. Training is an activity because time and other resources are invested in it. Each activity has a start and finish, signified by events. An activity begins with the completion of a prior event and ends with its own completion. In the PERT analysis, the project planning challenge is to enumerate all the critical activities of a project and to combine them into an efficient network structure, showing in what order the activities are to be performed.

It is of paramount importance to distinguish between activities in a sequential relationship and activities in a concurrent relationship. Two activities are in sequential relationship if one must be completed before the other can begin. For example, writing an advertisement must occur before placing that advertisement in a publication. Two activities are in a concurrent relationship if one can be completed independently of the other. Completing program documentation and obtaining approvals of copyright materials are in a concurrent relationship. The significance of this distinction is that project time can be cut down by making sure activities in a concurrent relationship are scheduled concurrently and not sequentially. This is especially true in a training environment.

A simplified PERT diagram is shown in Figure 6–4. This diagram is called a network planning diagram, a PERT diagram, or a critical path diagram. It portrays the events that must occur to complete a project. The events (shown in circles) are connected by arrows indicating "precedent" relationships. For example, event 6 cannot occur until events 4 and 5 are completed; event 5 cannot occur until event 2 is completed; event 4 cannot occur until events 2 and 3 are completed, and so on. Needless to say, this is a simple network. Construction of more complicated networks is greatly

F I G U R E   6–4

A Simplified PERT Diagram

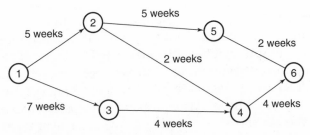

aided by today's personal computers and mainframe software programs. Indeed, networks can be constructed with unprecedented
ease and in a matter of minutes with programs such as SuperPro-
ject, Microsoft Project, and many others.

Every network contains several paths that define the possible
completion time of a project. A path through a network is a sequence of connected activities. In our simplified example in Figure
6–4, there are three paths: (a) 1,2,5,6; (b) 1,2,4,6; and (c) 1,3,4,6. The
first path is estimated to take 12 weeks, path 1,2,4,6 is estimated to
take 11 weeks, and path 1,3,4,6 is estimated to take 15 weeks. The
longest path through the network is called the critical path. The
length of the critical path corresponds to the minimum time required to complete the project. The last path is, therefore, considered the critical path. Since this path must be "traveled" and since
it consumes the greatest sum of time, it sets the earliest most likely
time for cooperation.

It should be noted that events along a noncritical path, such
as 1,2,5,6, can take place later than estimated without necessarily
delaying the 15-week estimated time for the project. In other
words, activities along noncritical paths have "slack" in their completion time.

The critical path is critical in two respects. First, any delays in
the actual time of completing any activity along the critical path
will delay the project by the amount of time of the delay. Second,
if the project manager finds the estimated completion time (in our
example, 15 weeks) to be too long, the critical path shows what
activities must be expected. (This means that the project manager

can shorten the duration of a critical activity and, hence, total project completion time, by investing more time, money, and people in it.)

Again, computations to find the best schedule are usually carried out on a personal computer or mainframe computer. With a mainframe computer, it takes approximately 30 seconds to find the time along the critical path for a project network of about 600 activities. PERT estimates the earliest time and latest time for each activity on a dated basis. Also, probability measures can be used to estimate the likelihood of completing any activity or the entire project in a given amount of time. Furthermore, computers make it convenient to "simulate" alternative networks and costs and to revise schedules from time to time.

The scheduling phase informs project team members when they may begin work and how much time is available to finish it. Some activities will be finished earlier than expected. Some activities because of uncontrollable events, and others because of neglect, will not be finished when expected. The discrepancies between actual times and estimated times will accumulate to the point when it may become necessary to reschedule the remaining activities. This is especially true when a project is moving slower than scheduled and there are penalties if the project is late.

The project manager may want to take corrective action in the form of "resource transfers" from slack activities to critical activities. Needless to say, control of a project is considerably facilitated by critical path analysis when used for updating and modifying the project's scheduling. In other words, critical path analysis (especially when used with a computer) shows the effect of different resource transfers on project completion time.

To make PERT effective, an information system is required to alert project managers when a project is being delayed. For more detailed information, see Kerzner (1995) and Haynes (1989).

FAILURE MODE AND EFFECT ANALYSIS

Failure mode and effect analysis (FMEA) is a systematic way to study the process and to determine and characterize the ways in which the service or product can fail. FMEA may be used in healthcare environments to identify known and potential problems before they occur and provide a priority for fixing them. For an extensive discussion on this topic, see Stamatis (1995).

REFERENCES

Brassard, M. *The Memory Jogger Plus*. Methuen, Mass.: GOAL/QPC, 1989.

Burr, J. T. *SPC: Tools for Operators*. Milwaukee: Quality Press, 1989.

Delbecq, A. L., and A. H. Van de Ven. *Group Techniques for Program Planning*. Middleton, Wis.: Green Briar Press, 1986.

Duncan, A. J. *Quality Control and Industrial Statistics*. 5th ed. Homewood, Ill.: Irwin, 1986.

Gitlow, H.; S. Gitlow; A. Oppenheim; and R. Oppenheim. *Tools and Methods for the Improvement of Quality*. Homewood, Ill.: Irwin, 1989.

Grant, E. L. and R. S. Leavenworth. *Statistical Quality Control*. 5th ed. New York: McGraw-Hill, 1980.

Gulezian, R. *Process Control Statistical Principles and Tools*. New York: Quality Alert Institute, 1991.

Haynes, M. E. *Project Management: From Idea to Implementation*. Los Altos, Calif.: Crisp Publications, 1989.

Improvement Tools. Miamisburg, Ohio: Productivity–Quality Systems, 1991.

Ishikawa K. *Guide to Quality Control*. White Plains, N.Y.: Kraus International Publications (Asian Productivity Organization), 1982.

Kerzner, H. *Project Management: A Systems Approach to Planning, Scheduling and Controlling*. 5th ed. New York: Van Nostrand Reinhold, 1995.

The Memory Jogger. Methuen, Mass.: GOAL/QPC, 1988.

Montgomery, D. C. *Introduction to Statistical Quality Control*. New York: John Wiley & Sons, 1985.

Shigeru, M. *Management for Quality Improvement: The 7 New QC Tools*. Cambridge, Mass.: Productivity Press, 1988.

Stamatis, D. H. *Failure Mode and Effect Analysis: From Theory to Execution*. Milwaukee: Quality Press, 1995.

CHAPTER 7

Advanced Topics of Quality

This chapter covers some selected advanced topics of quality as they relate to healthcare. We believe that the application of these topics to healthcare will help facilitate a smoother implementation of total quality management throughout the organization. The intent of the chapter is not to present an exhaustive study of the topics but rather to familiarize the reader with these concepts and provide some insight for the application to healthcare.

BENCHMARKING

Benchmarking is a tool, a technique or process, a philosophy, for determining "what to do, or goal setting," and "how to do it, or action plan identification." It can be applied systematically and comprehensively, as well as in an ad hoc project-by-project manner. It can require sophisticated statistical analysis, use of a wide variety of analytical tools, and a wide range of data sources. It usually requires time, effort, and resources. Also needed are a willingness to learn and to change, continuing long-term support by top management, an external focus on customers and competitors, a commonsense approach, active listening, and the ability to look at the old in a new way.

The term *benchmarking* was coined by Xerox in 1979. Since then, it has been used extensively in all kinds of industries with some startling results. In healthcare there is great opportunity to use benchmarking as a tool to compare or to find the best practices. Benchmarking may be the most important aspect of quality revolution in the making. It can provide data that can be used along with other systematic, comprehensive management approaches to improve performance. However, in no way, shape, or form is it an end unto itself. Benchmarking is a multidisciplinary effort.

In healthcare, benchmarking may be useful at different levels. From a broad management focus, benchmarking may result in cost reduction, profit improvement, business strategy development, total quality management implementation, and breakthrough opportunities. It also may benefit individual management processes, such as improving customer service, reducing product or service development time, market planning, and service/product distribution. When used from a highly specific focus, benchmarking may be instrumental in invoice design and in reduction of test costs and equipment failure.

Business Strategy Development

For a successful business strategy to be developed with benchmarking, an organization must decide which course it will follow. It must also be certain that it is realistically able to pursue that alternative. There are three areas of concern in identifying this strategy. They are:

1. Does an organization have the least cost? If so, what is the basis for the claim?

2. Is the organization differentiated in the eyes of the customer? If so, what is the basis for the claim?

3. How may competitive conditions change in the future?

Benchmarking can provide—at least in part—the information necessary to answer these concerns by providing focus and insight on what the best companies are doing. In addition to making a choice relative to least cost versus differentiation, an important strategy choice is that of being a mass marketer versus supplying the needs of your own specific market (e.g., laboratory and radiology services may be opened to the community as opposed to being used only for inpatients). For more information on generic strategies, see Higgins and Vincze (1989).

Characteristics of a Least Cost Strategy

A health organization following this strategy must be able to deliver a service with acceptable quality at a lower total cost than any of its competitors. Of special interest is the notion of total cost. Total cost is indeed the critical concern. The organization does not have to be least cost in every aspect of the business. Furthermore, the fact that the total cost is the lowest does not necessarily mean that the price it charges is the lowest. To determine if the least cost strategy is viable, it is necessary to perform competitive benchmarking and gain information relative to the following:

1. What is the relative market share of the company? Does the experience curve have a significant effect on cost reduction? (Where do we stand as an organization as far as the technology in all areas is concerned? Do we have the capital to sustain us in the investment of efficient systems?)

2. Do competitors have a different mix of fixed and variable costs?

3. What is the percent capacity utilization by competitive organizations?

4. Are the competitive firms using activity-based accounting?

5. How critical is raw material supply? Does our organization have preemptive sources of supply?

6. Does our organization have a tight system of budgeting and cost control for all functions?

7. Are services designed for low-cost production? Are services simplified and patient waiting lines reduced in number?

8. What is the level of service quality versus competition?

9. How labor intensive is your process? How effective are labor relations and management?

10. Are marginal accounts minimized?

Characteristics of a Differentiated Strategy

An organization following the differentiation strategy must be able to provide a unique product or service to meet the customer's expectations (see Chapter 1). It must be unique or different. The challenge to being unique is being able to provide a sustainable source of differentiation. It is difficult to create something that is totally sustainable. This may depend on a corporate culture producing a positive attitude toward quality and customer service or perhaps the value of information or computer-to-computer linkages.

Following a differentiation strategy does not mean that an organization can be inefficient relative to costs. Although cost is not the primary driving force, costs still must be minimized for the degree of differentiation provided. To determine if the differentiation strategy is viable, it is necessary to perform competitive benchmarking and gain information relative to the following:

1. Does the customer perceive something unique about the product or services provided? Is the customer willing to pay a premium price for this uniqueness?

2. What or who are the buying influences? What are the alternatives to the buying activity? What uniqueness does each of these value?

3. How has the competition differentiated itself and how does it position itself within the marketplace?

4. Does the organization have good marketing insights (information) that enable it to determine the basis for differentiation? Is this uniqueness brand image, technology, product/service features, before or after the sales service?

5. How important is company prestige, image, or brand loyalty in the buying decision?

6. Does the organization work harmoniously with various departments within the organization and with the suppliers and customer base?

7. Does the organization have the reputation and the compensation package required to attract and retain creative people?

For a detailed explanation, see Camp (1989, 1995), Stamatis (1995), and others.

QUALITY FUNCTION DEPLOYMENT

Quality function deployment (QFD) is a tool that was imported from Japan in the 1970s and is gaining momentum in just about every industry worldwide, including healthcare. In Japan, QFD is a means to translate the voice of the customer into design parameters that can be deployed horizontally through product planning, engineering, manufacturing, assembly, and service. However, QFD is much more than that. It is also a mechanism to identify conflicting requirements to be optimized and critical quality characteristics to be controlled through operational procedures.

The specific steps in QFD identify new quality technology and job functions necessary to carry out parameter deployment, which are clearly defined and assigned to particular individuals. For the organization benefit, QFD provides a historical reference to enhance future technology and to prevent errors from repeating themselves. Results are measured based on the number of changes during product or service development, time cycle to market, cost, and quality.

It is beyond the scope of the book to give an exhaustive explanation of QFD. For more information, see Akao (1990); Berwick, Godfrey, and Roessner (1991); Turner and Zipursky (1995); Nwabueze, Morris, and Haigh (1995); and American Supplier Institute (1987, 1989). However, a summary of QFD is appropriate. A good starting point to gain understanding of QFD involves two issues: voice of the customer and quality tables.

Voice of the Customer

Customers' needs, wants, and expectations expressed in their own words are original information, which often must be translated into technical language on the quality table (also known as the house of quality). If the customer is a manufacturer of industrial goods, that manufacturer can generally identify its own primary required quality characteristics. On the other hand, the buying public or a service recipient often mentions secondary or third-level requirements when asked what they want. For example, patients entering the hospital may say that what they want the most is to "get rid of the pain and suffering" and may say nothing about the competency of the physicians and staff or quality of the facilities. The funny part is, after discharge, the same patients may talk about specifics such as hospital food, safety issues, noise, and response time of the nurse. Because consumers' stated requirements often are incomplete, organizations must fill in the gaps revealed by the required quality matrix. The organizations often must work back from secondary or third-level requirements to primary ones.

Quality Tables

Various tables trace the way QFD is implemented in the stages of development and operation. These tables become very complicated, but their mission remains the same—to establish a systematic way of assigning responsibilities. These tables also serve to reveal potential bottlenecks. For example, the counterpart characteristics may set targets that conventional technology cannot attain.

Dealing with such bottlenecks is called bottleneck engineering, and developmental work must be concentrated on such a bottleneck.

QFD uses the design approach to break down the voice of the customer into segments and identifies specific means for achieving each segment. Its activities can be broken down into two fields: product/service quality deployment and deployment of quality function. Product/service quality deployment refers to the activities needed to convert customer-required quality, which may be fairly ill defined or incomplete, into specific quality characteristics. This process of conversion is defined as converting the customer requirements into counterpart characteristics, thus determining the design quality of the final product or service and, furthermore, systematically deploying the requirements to the quality of each task as well as functional components, in relation to process element.

The deployment of quality function refers to the activities needed to ensure that customer-required quality is achieved. This process is defined as deploying quality-related job functions step by step with both the series of objectives and means down to the finest detail. Even after counterpart quality characteristics have been set, each department must be assigned specific responsibilities. Otherwise, it will be difficult to ensure that the required quality will be achieved.

Steps of QFD

The approach to any QFD involves five steps:

1. *Customer requirements.* Finding out what the customer really needs, wants, and expects.
2. *Planning requirements.* Finding out what it will take to make the requirements workable.
3. *Design characteristics.* Finding out what are the basic customer quality requirements.
4. *Operational methods.* Finding out what it will take to incorporate these requirements into your working environment.
5. *Process sheets* (procedures). Implementing the changes and starting over again for further improvement.

Figure 7–1 shows a typical QFD timing schedule, and Figure 7–2 shows how the QFD methodology may be used in healthcare.

COST OF QUALITY

Cost of quality is the measurement of conformance and nonconformance to requirements set by the customer. It is the cost of poor quality or the wrong quality at work. Anytime the wrong things are done or things are done wrong, there is a cost to the organization. These costs can and do include rework, waste, unnecessary overtime, and job dissatisfaction. Participants will be able to estimate their organization's cost of quality, break down the cost of quality into avoidable costs and necessary costs, and plan how to reduce the avoidable costs of quality.

When we talk about cost of quality, we mean costs associated with the following: defects, mistakes, absenteeism, low morale, turf battles, confusion, late charges, inspection, scrap, grievances, retraining, duplication of effort, excess inventory, premium freight, overtime, rework, unnecessary field service, customer returns and allowances, lost time due to accidents, equipment failure, scheduling overlap, and many more.

The cost of quality is composed of two types of costs: (1) necessary and (2) avoidable (Figure 7–3). Necessary costs are required to achieve and sustain a defined standard of work. Avoidable costs occur whenever the wrong things are done or things are done the wrong way. Necessary costs include prevention and appraisal costs. Avoidable costs include some appraisal costs and failure costs. This relationship can be shown in the following quality grid:

---------------- **How you do it** ---------------->

Right Things Wrong	**Right Things Right**	
Delivered service as requested and on schedule, but incorrectly	Completed required report correctly and on schedule	(what you do)
Filled out correct form, but information was inaccurate	Provided requested service in an accurate, timely manner	
Wrong Things Wrong	**Wrong Things Right**	
Scheduled unnecessary, poorly run meeting	Ordered wrong equipment, but installed it correctly	
Sent bill to wrong person, and calculation was incorrect	Completed unnecessary but well-written report	

FIGURE 7-1

QFD Timing Schedule

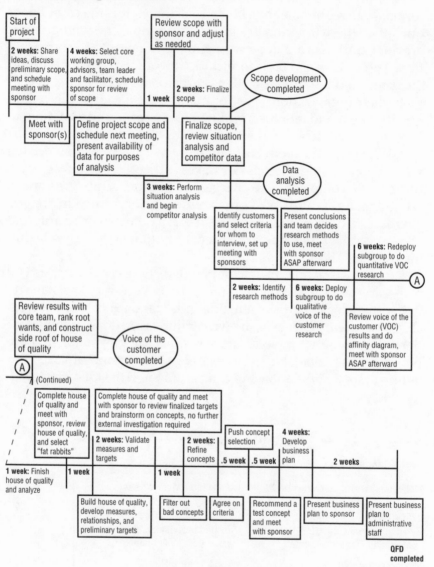

Employee's Role

The concept of doing "right things right" puts the responsibility for quality where it belongs—in the hands of each employee. Most employees have the potential to define what the right things are, but they can't do it alone. They must work with their customers and

FIGURE   7–2

QFD Development in Healthcare

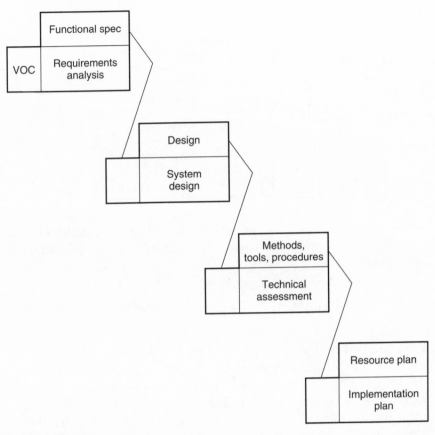

VOC indicates voice of the customer.

their supervisor to identify and understand customer and organizational needs. Employees can also determine how to do things right. Again, the employee does not operate in a vacuum. Quality is achieved only when the knowledge and skills of all employees are brought to bear on the work processes in which they are involved.

Manager's Role

In order to reduce the cost of quality, managers must communicate their priorities and expectations to their employees and facilitate the quality improvement process by involving employees and ensuring that they have the confidence and skill required to do the

FIGURE 7–3

Overall View of the Cost of Quality

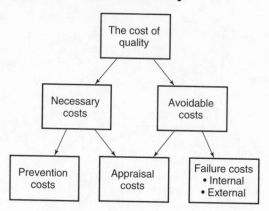

job. It is not the manager's job to provide solutions. Quality means that the best people to improve a work process are the people who do the work.

Prevention and Correction

The key to reducing costs and gaining the quality advantage is prevention. If a problem does occur, however, then the next best thing is early detection and treatment of the problem. For example, you might forget to add oil to your car. When you realize your oversight (perhaps not until the oil light goes on), you quickly remedy the situation. Your failure to do so would mean a large avoidable expense and the temporary loss of the use of your car. The best solution, however, is prevention. For example, you could set up a maintenance schedule for your car, which would include checking the oil on a regular basis. The same principle applies to problems in organizations. Prevention and early detection and correction of problems save time and money.

Price of Nonconformance

As a general rule, the cost of doing things wrong is associated with failing to maintain the standards of quality. As a consequence, these are the costs that must be controlled to minimize the overall cost of quality. These are the costs that an organization should fix and remove from the system, for example, the money spent for repair, rework, scrap/reject, and things that need to be done over again when they were not done correctly the first time. Our focus should be on identifying the correct way of doing the right things.

Price of Conformance

The costs of doing things correctly are associated with attaining and maintaining the specified quality set by the customer. Proper market research and product/service research and development will allow for the specifications or requirements to be developed to meet the needs and desires of the customer. Next, the product or service design must be developed to meet these stated requirements. Process development would also need to develop standards or requirements for product design to ensure that the product or service can be produced to meet the customer's requirements as described by the marketing and research activities.

When the product or the service design has been completed, process development would then develop the process or processes that would be required to meet the standards established for the specific product or service. Necessary methodology would next be designed and structured, which would satisfy the requirements of the customer and the product or service design. The cost of proper equipment, training, conforming supplies, proper facilities, and process verification would be a few of the more obvious examples of these items included in the price of conformance.

To monitor the processes, many techniques are available. One of the most common is the statistical process control (SPC) approach.

In healthcare the costs are not as easily identified nor quantified. They are hidden in day-to-day operation costs of the care provided. They include but are not limited to delays (both in scheduling and deliveries), business reputation, loss of future business, loss of market share, and a general negative customer attitude toward the service provided. These costs may even exceed what are considered the more tangible costs and may be more damaging to the sales of the company, since they are the items resulting directly from customer satisfaction.

When discussing quality and its effect on the costs of the organization, the final service or product of the company usually receives the exposure. Many of the costs associated with quality within the organization are in areas usually associated with the final product or service. However, if every job within the organization is considered to have an output, then quality of that job would become as important as the final product of the company. Each job has a set of requirements, suppliers, and customers. When each job output meets the requirements agreed to between the individual performing the job and the customer, it would be considered a quality job. An organization can lose considerable money as a result of not meeting these requirements and needing to do the task over again. Since the output of each job within the organization frequently is also the input to another, the costs can easily be compounded by causing another job to be done over again because of the failure of that input to meet the requirements. This can be as simple as the need to retype a letter because the writer did not take care to properly express the correct thought, or it could be as major as the need to redesign the Critical Care Unit because the nursing station was not hooked up properly with the patients' rooms and equipment.

The total cost of quality, the price of conformance plus the price of nonconformance, can generate very large cost numbers. In fact, from my experience in healthcare, these numbers run from 25 to 45 percent of revenues. What is interesting about these numbers, however, is the fact that the cost of quality is generated throughout the organization.

PROGRAMS FOR IMPROVING THE COST–QUALITY POSITION IN HEALTHCARE

The cost of quality has stirred much interest among healthcare executives. Competition from other healthcare organizations, governmental pressures, and other factors have pretty much forced the industry to evaluate all the things it is doing in an attempt to meet the cost of quality problem head on. Many programs are being instituted in numerous organizations whose purpose is to reduce the costs associated with quality or the lack of it. Among these programs are TQM, the Deming method of management, the Malcolm Baldrige National Quality Award (MBNQA) approach (see Chapter 9), and the ISO 9000 approach (see Chapter 8). All the methods depend on extensive education to provide the tools, motivation, and methods that the workers will need to recognize and solve problems.

These efforts to improve quality and reduce costs are all part of the struggle for survival that healthcare organizations are facing. Their success in improving quality and reducing costs will directly affect the ability of healthcare to survive. As their efforts imply, the survivability of healthcare organizations is related to competition, and the competition has been tied to the real or perceived quality of the products and services in the marketplace.

Once healthcare organizations recognize the relationship between cost and quality, the question is, What can we do about it? A number of programs can be instituted to reduce the cost of quality within an organization. However, it is of paramount importance to recognize that many of the programs are not a one-shot deal. They need the encouragement and support of management to make them part of the culture of the organization.

One technique which has been used with some success in manufacturing is participative management through team development. The workers are expected, with proper guidance and training, to develop the areas needing improvement, collect the necessary information, evaluate the problem and data, and propose solutions to the problems that affect their own work environment. Of course, this approach demands that management must be willing to accept some of the suggestions of the workers and develop a method to reward them for significant contributions.

Another approach to quality management does not place the emphasis on the workers but involves the entire company at all levels. The process of quality management is initiated when management realizes the need for action in the area of quality and becomes committed to doing something about it. Next, projections of the potential savings of the company, activity, or department are developed. Efforts are then focused to educate the entire department involved to ensure commonality of problem, language, tools, and expectations. The suppliers and the customers who need to participate in the process are active participants through focus groups, surveys, audits, interviews, and so on (whatever is applicable and appropriate).

Yet another approach is to depend on the financial department to evaluate your costs either with a standard cost approach or the newer approach of activity-based costing. Regardless of what method is used or to what extent, cost of quality is an important issue in the overall picture of the TQM concept and the welfare of the organization. A view of the effectiveness in the organization is shown in Figure 7–4.

DESIGN OF EXPERIMENTS

Design of experiments (DOE) is a way to find deeply hidden causes of process variation. DOE serves to break up variations into component parts and thus reveal primary causes. Another way of describing DOE is to say that the methodology helps to define the independent variables in such a way that the dependent variable is understood better by the experimenter. By understanding the relationship or relationships of dependent and independent variables, we can modify, adjust, or even completely change the process. We can fix (current) or improve (current and future) or predict (future) the process.

By using DOE in the healthcare industry, it is possible to study the effects of several variables at one time and to study interrelationships and interactions. DOE techniques are useful for deliberately disturbing causes usually in balance, breaking apart effects of hidden variables, and studying possible effects of variables during service (process) design, development, or implementation.

Experiments in processes range from informal changes introduced randomly to carefully planned, highly structured experiments. To study these changes, we use three principal approaches: the classical, Taguchi, and Shainin methods. All of them have advantages and disadvantages. The appropriate method depends on the application and the understanding of the method and the process by the experimenter. However, regardless of the method used, this sequence is followed:

I. Experiment
    A. Statement of the problem
    B. Choice of response or dependent variable
    C. Selection of factors to be varied

F I G U R E   7–4

A Diagram of Cost of Quality over Time

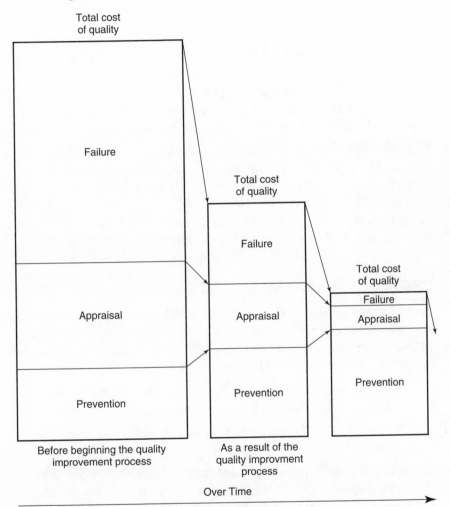

D. Choice of levels of these factors
   1. Quantitative or qualitative
   2. Fixed or random
E. How factor levels are to be combined

II. Design
  A. Number of observations to be taken
  B. Order of experimentation
  C. Method of randomization to be used
  D. Mathematical model to describe the experiment
  E. Hypothesis to be tested
III. Analysis
  A. Data collection and processing
  B. Computation of test statistics
  C. Interpretation of results for the experimenter

It is beyond the scope of this book to address the details of even a typical DOE. However, the reader is encouraged to see Hicks (1982); Dayton (1970); Peace (1993); Bhote (1991); Cohen and Cohen (1983); Roy (1990); Ross (1988); Cox and Snell (1981); Taguchi (1987); Lehmann (1986); Rousseeuw and Leroy (1987); and Box, Hunter, and Hunter (1978) for explanation and applications.

PROJECT MANAGEMENT

Project management is the application of knowledge, skills, tools, and techniques to meet or exceed stakeholder requirements from a project. Meeting or exceeding stakeholder requirements means balancing competing demands among the following:

- Scope, time, cost, quality, and other project objectives.
- Stakeholders with differing requirements.
- Identified requirements and unidentified requirements (expectations).

In healthcare, project management may play an important role in the implementation of TQM throughout the organization. One of the reasons that project management may be important is the fact that TQM and its implementation may be seen as a project. We all know that organizations perform work, and work generally involves either operations or projects (although the two may overlap). Operations and projects share many characteristics. For example they are performed by people; constrained by limited resources; able to be described as processes and subprocesses; and planned, executed, and controlled. They differ primarily in that operations are ongoing and repetitive while projects are temporary and unique. A project can thus be defined in terms of its distinctive characteristics; it is a temporary endeavor undertaken to create a unique product or service. Temporary means that every project has a definite ending point. Unique means the product or service is different in some distinguishing way from all similar products or services.

The reader must be careful here not to confuse the concept of TQM with the implementation of TQM. The two are not the same. The concept of TQM is a philosophy; therefore, it is perpetual. On the other hand, the implementation of TQM is indeed a project with a definite beginning and hopefully a definite end (Stamatis 1994). For a detailed discussion of the TQM implementation using project management, see Stamatis (1995). For additional information on project management, see Kerzner (1995); Geddes, Hastings, and Briner (1990); and Lock (1994).

MEASUREMENT

How much air did you breathe today? How many calories are there in a candy bar? How far is it to the moon? How large is the tumor? How much light is needed for you to read this page? All these questions can be answered by measurements. The food we eat, the water we drink, and the air we breathe have been measured. Light, heat, electricity, and sound have been measured. Perhaps your eyesight, your intelligence, or your running speed also has been measured.

What is meant by measurement? How are things measured? Who invented the units used to measure things? How do we compute in measured quantities? These are questions you need to know if you are going to use measuring principles appropriately and accurately. Basically, a measurement associates a number with some unit of measure in order to describe some property of a person or thing. When we talk about measurements, we must keep things and their properties separate. "Things" are natural objects such as boxes, football, or human beings. The property of things refers to characteristics such as color, length, volume, temperature, pressure, weight, or intelligence. We *always* measure the properties, *not* the things. We do not measure a boy named Cary; we measure Cary's weight, temperature, or height. In this way, measurement gives us information. To describe Cary as being 6 feet 2 inches tall gives more information than to say Cary is a tall boy.

An important part of measurement is the unit of measure. For example, we use inches or centimeters for dimensions, quarts or liters for fluids, pounds or kilograms for weight, and so on. When we measure a quantity, we find how many of the appropriate units of measure it contains.

History of Measurement

The history of humans is, in part, a history of measurement. Measurement started by comparing things. By comparison, early humans were able to determine that one herd of animals was larger than another. When numbers were developed, this comparison was made by counting. Later, better units of measure were developed. And even later, these measurements became standardized. In the process of accomplishing standardization of measurements, we developed standard measuring scales, precision measuring instruments, and a system for computing in measured quantities essential parts of a useful system of measures. The result of all this is that measurement is a combination of mathematics, science, and mechanics, working in tandem to create a better understanding of the property of things. As mathematics, science, and mechanics have improved, measurements have also improved.

In healthcare we see measurement in all areas of the industry: in hospitals, private practices of physicians, laboratories, pharmacies, and so on. In fact, without measurement, healthcare would be in real trouble. Measurement in healthcare allows the system to identify its own present state, compare it to something else (standard or competition), and then monitor its movement (stability, improvement, or even deterioration)

Precision of Measurement

The measuring instrument we use to make a measurement depends on what we are measuring. For example, a thermometer is used to measure temperature, not air pressure. The measuring instrument we use might also depend on the size of the measurement we are making. We use odometers, not rulers, to measure the distance between two towns. The scale or the dial on a measuring device is usually marked off to measure units or fractions of units. A ruler, for instance, may be marked off into millimeters. The smaller the unit or fraction of a unit that a device can measure, the more precisely it will measure. The precision of a measurement, then, depends on the size of the unit of measure used to make it. The smaller the unit of measurement, the more precise the measurement. A scale that is marked to give readings in grams is much more accurate than the scale that is marked in kilograms.

Accuracy of Measurement

Although two recorded measurements may have the same precision, the size of the absolute error may be more important in one than in the other. An error of 1 milligram may not be important in measuring one food serving, but it would be very serious in prescribing a specific medication. The accuracy of a measurement is always given in terms of the relative error. The smaller the relative error, the greater the accuracy of the measurement. Remember that the precision of a measurement is determined by the absolute error and the accuracy by the relative error where: absolute error is the greatest possible error of the measurement, and relative error is absolute error/recorded measurement.

CAPABILITY STUDIES
Control versus Specifications

A process is said to be operating in statistical control when only sources of variation are common causes. The primary function of a process control system is to provide a statistical signal when special causes of variation are present, and so to enable appropriate action that can eliminate those causes and prevent their reappearance. See Figures 5–8 and 7–5.

Process capability is determined by the total variation that comes from common causes—the minimum variation that can be achieved after all special causes have been eliminated. Thus, capability represents the performance potential of the process itself, as demonstrated when the process is being operated in a state of statistical control. Capability is usually measured by the proportion of output that will be within specification tolerances. Since a process in statistical control can be described as a predictable distribution, capability can be expressed in terms of this distribution, and the proportion of out-of-specification items can be realistically evaluated. If this is excessive, actions to reduce the variation from common causes will be required to make the process capable of consistently meeting the specification.

In short, the process must first be brought into statistical control (see Figure 7–5a) so its performance can be predicted; then its capability to meet specifications can be assessed. Before we pursue process capability, it is of paramount importance to understand the

FIGURE 7–5

A Process in Control and out of Control

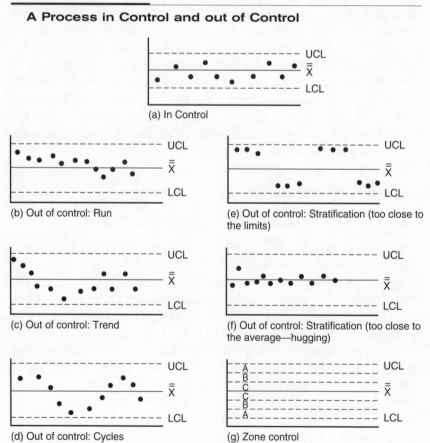

(a) In Control

(b) Out of control: Run

(c) Out of control: Trend

(d) Out of control: Cycles

(e) Out of control: Stratification (too close to the limits)

(f) Out of control: Stratification (too close to the average—hugging)

(g) Zone control

difference between control limits and specifications. The difference is that control limits are calculated numbers based on the process itself, whereas specifications are given to you by the customer (see Figure 5–8).

Capability

Capability is the spread of performance of a process in a state of statistical control—the amount of variation from common causes identified after all special causes of variation have been eliminated. Capability can be expressed in several ways, for example, (1) the values within which a given proportion of output will fall; (2) the proportion of output that falls within given values; and (3) in terms of indexes, that is, capability ratio (Cr), process capability (Cp), or Cpk.

Having determined that a process is in statistical control, the question still remains whether the process is capable, namely, is its performance to specification acceptable? If the capability is not acceptable, then an important shift will have to be made in seeking improvement actions, since capability reflects variation from common causes, which almost always represents system faults that require management action to correct.

The procedure to assess process capability begins after control issues reflected in both the average and range charts have been resolved (special causes identified, analyzed, corrected, and prevented from recurring) and the ongoing control charts reflect a process that is in statistical control preferably for 25 or more subgroups (usually each subgroup has three to five samples apiece). This involves comparing the distribution of the process output with the engineering specifications, to see whether the specifications can consistently be met.

There are several techniques for assessing the capability of a process that is in statistical control. Most of them assume normality (a bell-shaped normal distribution). If it is not known whether the distribution is normal, a test for normality should be made. If nonnormality is suspected or confirmed, more flexible techniques should be used, such as computerized curve-fitting or graphical analysis–probability graph paper analysis.

It is beyond the scope of this book to explain the capability techniques available to the practitioner. However, the reader may see Grant and Leavenworth (1980), Gitlow et al. (1989), Gulezian (1991), and Montgomery (1985) for extensive reading on this issue.

REPEATABILITY AND REPRODUCIBILITY STUDIES

Is there a need to worry about measurement, reproducibility, repeatability, accuracy, precision and so on in healthcare? One may discard this section as superfluous; however, remember that everything in healthcare involves measurement. The question then is not whether repeatability and reproducibility are appropriate topics of discussion but how detailed we want to get in the process of measurement. For example, in the lab, how do we know that the hematology machine is operating at an acceptable level? Or how do we know if the breathing machine is capable of operating at the levels prescribed by the respiratory physician?

Our focus then in performing a measurement analysis is to identify as much as possible where the variation is coming from and to what extent this variation is affecting our outcome. The analysis is based on percent of tolerance or percent of variation, with the following guidelines for acceptance.

Error	Guideline
< 10%	Measurement system is OK
10–30%	May be acceptable based on importance of application, cost of measurement system, cost of repairs, etc.
> 30%	Measurement system needs improvement; make every effort to identify and correct problems

Measurement studies should be performed wherever there is an instrument that needs calibration and processes that need validation. The two most important ingredients of this analysis are repeatability and reproducibility. For more information, see Montgomery (1985) and Automotive Industry Action Group (1990).

Repeatability

Repeatability of the measurement process implies the gauge variability itself is consistent. Two sources of repeatability errors are measurement variations due to the gauge itself and positional variation of the item in the gauge. Since both of these variations are represented by the subgroup ranges of repeated measurements, the range chart will show the consistency of the measurement process. If the range chart is out of control, there is generally a problem with the consistency of the measurement process. Those points identified as out of control should be investigated for their special cause of inconsistency and corrected.

Reproducibility

Reproducibility of the measurement process implies operator variability itself is consistent. One way to think of operator variability is that it represents the incremental bias that can be attributed to each operator. If this bias or operator variability does exist, the individual operators' overall averages will differ. This can be seen on the average control chart by comparing the operator averages for each part. The operator variation or reproducibility is estimated by determining the overall average for each operator and then finding the range by subtracting the smallest operator average from the largest.

Short Method Repeatability and Reproducibility Study

Another method combines repeatability and reproducibility. To conduct this study, two requirements are necessary: accuracy and repeatability and reproducibility.

Accuracy
Have one operator measure the same item 10 times and a standard 10 times. Average the readings from each. The difference between the averages is the inaccuracy or bias.

Repeatability and Reproducibility
To conduct this phase of the study, there are six steps:

    1. Randomly select and number five items.

    2. Two operators each measure the parts and record them in a row corresponding to the part. Place the results on a format similar to Table 7–1.

3. The difference in reading is recorded as range—no negative numbers here.

4. Calculate the average range—R bar.

5. RR error = (R bar/D-2) × (5.15). (This will account for 99 percent of the normal distribution.) The value of 5.15 is always constant, and the value for D-2 is found in Table 7–2.

6. Divide RR error by the tolerance and multiply by 100 percent.

TABLE 7–1

Typical Form for Placing Operator Information

Parts	Operator A	Operator B	Range
1			
2			
3			
4			
5			
Sum of ranges			
Average range			

TABLE 7–2

D-2 Values for Distribution of R Bar

Parts	Operator 2	Operator 3
1	1.41	1.91
2	1.28	1.81
3	1.23	1.77
4	1.21	1.75
5	1.19	1.74

REFERENCES

Akao, Y., ed. *Quality Function Deployment*. Cambridge, Mass.: Productivity Press, 1990.

American Supplier Institute. *Quality Function Deployment*. Dearborn, Mich.: American Supplier Institute, 1987.

————. *Transactions from a Symposium on Quality Function Deployment*. Dearborn, Mich.: American Supplier Institute, 1989.

Automotive Industry Action Group. *Measurement Systems Analysis: Reference Manual*. Southfield, Mich.: Automotive Industry Action Group, 1990.

Berwick, D. M.; A. B. Godfrey; and J. Roessner. *Curing Healthcare*. San Francisco: Jossey Bass, 1990.

Bhote, K. R. *World Class Quality*. New York: AMACOM, 1991.

Box, G. E. P.; W. G. Hunter; and J. S. Hunter. *Statistics for Experimenters*. New York: John Wiley & Sons, 1978.

Camp, R. C. *Benchmarking: The Search for Industry Best Practices That Lead to Superior Performance*. Milwaukee, Wisc.: Quality Press, 1989.

Camp, R. C. *Business Process Benchmarking: Finding and Implementing Best Practices*. Milwaukee, Wisc.: Quality Press, 1995.

Cohen, J., and P. Cohen. *Applied Multiple Regression/Correlation Analysis for the Behavioral Sciences*. 2d ed. Hillsdale, N.J.: Lawrence Erlbaum Associates, 1983.

Cox, D. R., and E. J. Snell. *Applied Statistics*. New York: Chapman & Hall, 1981.

Dayton, C. M. *The Design of Educational Experiments*. New York: McGraw-Hill, 1970.

Geddes, M.; C. Hastings; and W. Briner. *Project Leadership*. Hampshire, England: Ashridge Management College, 1990.

Gitlow, H.; S. Gitlow; A. Oppenheim; and R. Oppenheim. *Tools and Methods for the Improvement of Quality*. Homewood, Ill.: Irwin, 1989.

Grant, E. L., and R. S. Leavenworth. *Statistical Quality Control*. 5th ed. New York: McGraw-Hill, 1980.

Gulezian, R. *Process Control: Statistical Principles and Tools*. New York: Quality Alert Institute, 1991.

Hall, W. K. "Survival Strategies in a Hostile Environment." *Harvard Business Review*, September–October 1980, pp. 54–62.

Hicks, C. R. *Fundamental Concepts in the Design of Experiments*. New York: Holt, Rinehart & Winston, 1982.

Higgins, H., and R. Vincze. *Strategic Management:* New York: Dryden Press, 1989, p. 176.

Kerzner, H. *Project Management: A Systems Approach to Planning, Scheduling and Controlling*. 5th ed. New York: Van Nostrand Reinhold, 1995.

Lehmann, E. L. *Testing Statistical Hypotheses*. 2d ed. New York: John Wiley & Sons, 1986.

Lock, D., ed. *Handbook of Project Management*. 2d ed. Hampshire, England: Gower Technical Press, 1994.

Montgomery, D. C. *Statistical Quality Control*. New York: John Wiley & Sons, 1985.

Nwabueze, U.; D. S. Morris; and R. H. Haigh. "Organizational Diagnosis: A Healthcare Experience of BPR." In *ASQC 49th Annual Quality Congress Proceedings*. Milwaukee: American Society of Quality Control, 1995, pp. 833–39.

Peace, G. S. *Taguchi Methods: A Hands-On Approach*. Reading, Mass.: Addison-Wesley, 1993.

Ross, P. J. *Taguchi Techniques for Quality Engineering*. New York: McGraw-Hill, 1988.

Rousseeuw, P. J., and A. M. Leroy. *Robust Regression and Outlier Detection*. New York: John Wiley & Sons, 1987.

Roy, R. *A Primer on the Taguchi Method*. New York: Van Nostrand Reinhold, 1990.

Stamatis, D. H. "Total Quality Management and Project Management." *Project Management Journal*, September 1994, pp. 48–54.

————. *Total Service Quality*. Delray Beach, Fla.: St. Lucie Press, 1995.

Taguchi, G. *System of Experimental Design*. Vols. 1 & 2. White Plains, N.Y.: Kraus International Publications, 1987.

Turner, R. B., and L. S. Zipursky. "Quality Tools Help Improve Employee Commitment." In *ASQC 49th Annual Quality Congress Proceedings*. Milwaukee: American Society for Quality Control, 1995, pp. 770–76.

CHAPTER 8

ISO 9000 Standards and Healthcare

This chapter deals with the quality standards document known as the ISO 9000 and its relationship to healthcare. Specifically, it covers the definition of the ISO, its development and purpose, the benefits, and the certification process. The intent of this chapter is not to give an exhaustive explanation of the topic, as other full-length books have been written about it. For detailed information, see Peach (1994), Stamatis (1995), and Lamprecht (1992).

PURPOSE OF ISO

Since 1987 the international community has standardized some of the issues of quality in what has come to be known as the ISO 9000 standards. The essence of the standard is to define quality at its most common denominator in all industries and to provide some assurance of consistency. Actually, the ISO 9000 standards are a bundle of standards, which include the following:

ISO 9000-1: A set of guidelines for the selection and use of the appropriate standards ISO 9001, 9002, and 9003.

ISO 9001: A model for quality assurance for companies involved in the design and development, production, installation, and servicing of a product or service. There are 20 elements in this standard.

ISO 9002: A model for quality assurance for companies involved only in the production, installation, and servicing of a product. There are 19 elements in this standard.

ISO 9003: A model for quality assurance for companies involved in final inspection and testing. There are 16 elements in this standard.

ISO 9004-1: A guide for the application of the various elements of the quality management system.

DEFINITION OF ISO

The ISO in ISO 9000 is not, as generally assumed, the acronym for the International Organization for Standardization. Rather, it is the Greek word meaning "equal." How fitting, since the intent of the standards is to harmonize the world of quality globally. In fact, as of this writing, more than 90 countries have agreed to follow these standards. The United States is represented through the American National Standards Institute (ANSI). The objective of the ISO is to promote the development of standards worldwide for purposes of improved operating efficiency, improved productivity, and reduced cost.

HISTORY OF ISO

In 1959 the U.S. Department of Defense established a quality management program under the designation MIL-Q-9858. Four years later the program was revised (MIL-Q-9858A), and then in 1968 NATO essentially adopted the provisions of MIL-Q-9858A in its Allied Quality Assurance Publication 1 (AQAP-1). In 1970 the Ministry of Defense in the United Kingdom incorporated most of the provisions of AQAP-1 in its Management Program Defense Standard, DEF/STAN 05-8. Recently DEF/STAN 05-8 has been modified to reflect the provisions of ISO 9000 and has taken on the designation DEF/STAN 05–21, 22, 23, and 24 to align itself with ISO 9001, 9002, 9003, and 9004.

In 1979 the British Standards Institute developed the first commercial Quality Management System standards from these predecessors, which became known as BS 5750. In 1987 the International Organization for Standardization created the ISO 9000 standards, which adopted most of the elements of BS 5750. In that same year, BS 5750 and ISO 9000 were harmonized to make them equivalent documents. Also in that same year, the European Community—presently known as the European Union—adopted this harmonized set of standards and designated it EN (European Norme) 9000. Finally, in 1987, the American Society for Quality Control (ASQC) and the American National Standards Institute (ANSI) established and published what is now called the Q 9000 series, which is basically the ISO 9000 standard except with some differences in terminology. Even though the two standards officially have different names, they are equivalent.

ISO CONTENTS

The standards cover a wide range of activities for the entire organization, as can be seen in Table 8–1. The table shows the content of each element and the content of each standard.

The 1994 Changes

Like everything else, change occurs even in the ISO standards. The latest changes occurred in 1994 and they had more of a clarifying nature to the existing elements rather than adding more items. In any case, the standards have a formal review cycle of five years, at which time adjustments and new changes become part of the standard. The 1994 changes from the original 1987 ISO 9000 series are summarized as follows:

1. The role of management is enhanced and emphasized.
2. ISO 9002 now includes servicing (4.19), and all the elements have been renumbered to reflect agreement with the ISO 9001. Element 4.4 (design) is marked N/A.
3. The word *customer* has displaced the original word of *purchaser.*
4. Quality policy is required to be closely related with the customer's needs, wants, and expectations as well as management's objectives.
5. ISO 9003 has been greatly expanded to include everything in ISO 9001 except design, purchasing, process control, and servicing.

T A B L E   8–1

Hierarchy of ISO Standards, Their Elements, and Their Contents

Standard	Element	Description
ISO 9001	4.4	Design and research and development
ISO 9002	4.19	Servicing
	4.9	Process control
	4.6	Purchasing
ISO 9003	4.20	Statistical techniques
	4.18	Training
	4.17	Quality audits
	4.16	Quality records
	4.15	Handling, storage, packaging, preservation, and delivery
	4.14	Corrective and preventive action
	4.13	Control of nonconforming product
	4.12	Inspection and test status
	4.11	Inspection, measuring, and test equipment
	4.10	Inspection and testing
	4.8	Product identification and traceability
	4.7	Control of customer-supplied product
	4.5	Document control
	4.3	Contract review
	4.2	Quality system
	4.1	Management responsibility

6. A quality manual now is a requirement.

7. Quality planning receives a greater emphasis in the quality system either as a stand alone or as a standard activity of the overall system.

8. Contract amendments receive specific mention.

9. Design reviews are now mandatory.

10. The confusion of "verification of purchased product" has been eliminated.

11. The requirement of process control (4.9) has been expanded to include the maintenance of equipment.

12. ISO 10012 is identified as a guidance document in connection with calibration.

13. Preventive action is added to element 4.14 and is distinguished from corrective action.

14. ISO 10011 now becomes a formal guide for the management of audits (training, conduct, and internal audits).

15. Identification of the need for statistical techniques is now a stated requirement.

GROWTH OF ISO

The ISO 9000 standards have become very prevalent in many industries. However, when the dust settles and the frenzy is over, we will recognize that the thrust for the ISO 9000 success story is that it has become purely a market-driven item. The customer has become such a driving force that, in the European Union, officials are currently discussing mandatory regulatory requirements relative to certification and registration. This is especially true in regulated industries, such as the medical products and telecommunications industries.

Moreover, there is growth toward universal acceptance of ISO 9000 as a true international standard. ISO 9000 quality management system standards have been adopted by the U.K. Ministry of Defense and by NATO. The U.S. Department of Defense now permits the use of ISO 9000 systems on contracts. The U.S. Food and Drug Administration has also incorporated ISO 9000 requirements in its proposed revision of GMP (good manufacturing practice) standards for medical devices.

Quality management systems are an essential element of such initiatives as total quality management and the Malcolm Baldrige National Quality Award. The ISO quality management system is indeed an ideal candidate for adoption in the healthcare industry, given its growing recognition and acceptance as well as the dire need for reform in the industry at large.

BENEFITS OF ISO IN HEALTHCARE

There are many benefits related to the ISO system certification and registration process, not all of them associated with international recognition and registration in a directory. Perhaps two of the most important benefits in healthcare are improved quality and productivity. As stated earlier, ISO 9000 certification ensures a higher level of product or service quality and productivity through an unbiased independent professional assessment and evaluation against a standard whose elements address some of the most fundamental building blocks of good management. This goal is accomplished largely through the assurance that a good, sound quality management system exists and is functioning properly.

Another benefit of ISO in healthcare is reduction of cost. If the quality management system has been implemented and is working effectively, many costs associated with rework, repair, reject/scrap, and inefficiency will be reduced or eliminated. The quality management system focuses its attention on the process of problem prevention in the interest of saving time and labor.

APPLICABILITY OF ISO IN HEALTHCARE

To be sure, the ISO was originally designed for manufacturing businesses. However, since its acceptance by so many so fast, the International Organization for Standardization (1991) has issued a guideline for services (ISO 9004-2), which explains the transition from manufacturing to service. There are some points to overcome, especially in the terminology domain, but nothing should prevent a healthcare organization from receiving an ISO 9000 certification.

A case in point is a private hospital in the United Kingdom that achieved registration to ISO 9002, illustrating the relevance of the series to an increasingly wide range of organizations. The 50-bed BUPA Cambridge Lea Hospital became the first surgical hospital in the country to have its quality assurance system registered. The hospital already had a reputation for quality; however, this could not be proved. It was decided by management that an independent authority would remedy this. The remedy for such recognition was the ISO 9002. Achieving certification to ISO 9002 would give the hospital a marketing edge over its rivals, not only in the United Kingdom but throughout the world.

The decision to proceed with ISO 9000 implementation was taken in March 1992. A quality system was already in place, but this had to be documented fully to meet the standard. Therefore, appropriate quality manuals, procedures, instructions, and supported records had to meet the requirements of the standard. To be sure, the hospital had a few difficulties in translating what is, in effect, a standard for the manufacturing industry into something that is meaningful in a healthcare environment. Much interpretation was required. The standard's term *process control* became *patient care*, for example. Final inspection and testing became patient discharge, and inspection and test status became patient records.

To prepare for assessment, the hospital employed someone with ISO 9000 experience on a six-month contract to prepare documentation. A consultant also was brought in to provide internal audit training and to go through a preassessment audit. The BUPA Cambridge Lea Hospital was assessed by the British Standards Institution Quality Assurance in January 1993. Other hospitals in the BUPA group will be attempting ISO 9000 registration over the next few years.

It is too early to say what the long-term benefits are, but many improvements have been identified. All the staff members are proud to be at the first surgical hospital in the United Kingdom to achieve ISO 9002 certification. As a result of undertaking ISO 9000, there is undoubtedly greater staff involvement in all quality issues and an increase in awareness of other people's roles in other parts of the hospital. It has made the staff members aware that they can start the change process and that maintaining high standards is everyone's responsibility.

CERTIFICATION PROCESS

The ISO certification process involves on-site assessment and subsequent registration. It can be divided into four stages:

1. *Determination of readiness.* At the first stage the organization seeking assessment for certification is tested for its readiness. This readiness involves a brief evaluation relative to the constituent elements required by the ISO 9000 process. If the organization is ready, it can proceed directly to the assessment stage by submitting an application for certification. If not, it can seek preparation or consultant services to pave the way for successful assessment and certification.

2. *Preparation services.* This is the stage when policies, procedures, instructions, and so on are prepared in a formal way for compliance to the standard. This preparation may be performed by representatives of the organization or outside consultants or both. Most of the problems identified at this stage have to do with documentation control, design control, purchasing, inspection, and test and process control.

3. *Documentation review and assessment* (on site). The documentation review of the quality system is performed to determine its adequacy for assessment. This is typically done six to eight weeks before the planned assessment date, to give the organization time to overcome any minor noncompliance problems. The actual assessment takes no more than one to two weeks and assesses the effectiveness of the system.

4. *Assessment, review, and registration.* At the final stage, typically the assessment is reviewed against the established criteria of the appropriate ISO 9000 standard and a determination is made whether any noncompliances exist. If so, corrective action must be pursued, and time is given objectively to demonstrate that the problems have indeed been fixed. That usually takes 30 to 60 days. If there are no noncompliances, the certification is issued, and the organization is registered as an ISO 9000 certified organization.

The average length of time for certification ranges from 15 to 24 months depending on the status of the organization seeking certification. Once the certification has been issued, the registrar must perform a semiannual audit to make sure that the organization stays in compliance. This semiannual audit is a much shorter assessment than the original and focuses on selected elements of the standard, corrective action, use of the certification logo, and past problem areas.

REFERENCES

International Organization for Standardization. *ISO 9004-2: Quality Management and Quality System Elements—Part 2: Guidelines for Services.* Geneva, Switzerland: International Organization for Standardization, 1991.

Lamprecht, J. L. *ISO 9000 Preparing for Registration.* New York: Marcel Dekker and Milwaukee: Quality Press, 1992.

Peach, R. W., ed. *The ISO 9000 Handbook.* 2nd ed. Fairfax, Va.: CEEM Information Services, 1994.

Stamatis, D. H. *ISO 9000 Implementation and Understanding the Basic Blocks to Quality.* New York: Marcel Dekker, 1995.

CHAPTER 9

Malcolm Baldrige National Quality Award and Healthcare

This chapter will address the Malcolm Baldrige National Quality Award (MBNQA) and how it relates to healthcare. Specifically, it will review the historical background of the award and define each of its categories. A cursory analysis of the award process also is provided. This review is based on U.S. Department of Commerce (1995), Stamatis (1995), Heaphy and Gruska (1995), and Nordeen (1991).

HISTORY

The Malcolm Baldrige National Quality Award was created by Public Law 100-107 and was signed into law on August 20, 1987. The award program led to the creation of a new public–private partnership. Principal support for the program comes from the foundation for the Malcolm Baldrige National Quality Award, established in 1988. The award is named for Malcolm Baldrige, who served as U.S. Secretary of Commerce from 1981 until his death in a rodeo accident in 1987. His managerial excellence contributed to long-term improvement in efficiency and effectiveness of government.

MBNQA PRINCIPLES

It has been said that the award is truly a quality approach for organizations to follow if they are committed to quality excellence and/or world-class competition. The essence of the MBNQA is contained in the following 10 points:

1. Quality is defined by the customer: Quality is judged by the customer. The customer's expectations of quality dictate product or service design, and this, in turn, drives the organization. All product and service attributes that lead to customer satisfaction and preference must be taken into consideration. The MBNQA views the customer-driven quality as a strategic concept.

2. The senior management of a business needs to have clear quality values and build the values into the way the company operates on a day-to-day basis. A company's senior management must create clear quality values, specific goals, and well-defined systems and methods for achieving the goals. Ongoing personal involvement is essential. The attitude must be changed from management control to management committed to help you. In other words, leadership is a critical issue in the organization.

3. Quality excellence derives from well-designed and well-executed systems and processes. Criteria design requirements must meet high standards, be clear, have a diagnostic potential, meet international standards, and be able to communicate the essentials of the design.

4. Continuous improvement must be part of the management of all systems and processes. Constant improvement in many directions is required. Some examples are improved products and services, reduced errors and defects, improved responsiveness, and improved efficiency and effectiveness in the use of resources.

5. Companies need to develop goals, as well as strategic and operational plans, to achieve quality leadership. Two terms that are used interchangeably are *objective* and *goal*. There is, of course, no one right definition. As long as the terms are used consistently within an organization, it does not really matter which term is preferred. For our purposes, *objectives* are broad areas in which something is to be accomplished, for example, customer service. *Goals* are specific and measurable and have a time frame, for example, bill all Medicaid invoices within 33 days by the end of September 1996. For best results, goals should be attainable, fair, challenging, and effective. At the same time, we must differentiate between result goals and effort goals. Result goals define the specific performance measure to be achieved, whereas effort goals define specific accomplishments that are completely under the control of the goal setter.

The decisions made regarding goals can have a profound interaction with the mission statement of the company and the values as defined in the statement of guiding principles. Because of the importance that goals have in the organization, we must also recognize their structure. There are two structures: (a) the cascading goal structure and (b) the interdepartmental goal. The cascading goal structure is a consistent goal structure that provides focus and direction to the entire organization. To create this, start with the most important goal, as viewed by the administrator or chief operating officer, and decompose each of these by functional area working from one management level to the next. For example, starting with a return on equity goal, what does this mean that each department has to do? What does this suggest in the way of specific contributions?

Interdepartmental goals are the most elusive goals in the organization, primarily because it is very difficult to get all the departments to work together toward a common set of goals. One way to manage this is to have each department indicate its goals and what it requires in the way of performance from other departments to reach those goals. A cross-tabulation can then be used to develop the total goals for a department or function.

6. An effort to shorten the response time of all company operations and processes needs to be part of quality improvement. There is an increasing need for shorter new product and service development and introduction cycles and a more rapid response to customers.

7. Operations and decisions of the company need to be based on facts and data. A wide range of facts and data are required, for example, customer satisfaction, competitive evaluations, supplier data, and data relative to internal operations. Performance indicators to track operational and competitive performance are critical. These performance indicators or goals can act as the cohesive or unifying force within an organization. They can also provide the basis for recognition and reward.

8. All employees must be suitably trained and involved in quality activities. Reward and recognition systems need to reinforce total participation and the emphasis on quality. Factors bearing on the safety, health, and well-being of employees need to be included in the improvement objectives. Effective training is required. The emphasis must be on preventing mistakes, not merely correcting them. Employees must be trained to have responsibility for (inspect) their own work on a continuous basis.

9. Design quality and prevention of defects and errors should be major elements of the quality system. It is of paramount importance that the organization have a system of prevention that is effective and documented. Furthermore, there should exist a feedback system for corrective action for items that do not make the quality standards as the organization has defined them.

10. Companies need to communicate quality requirements to suppliers and work with suppliers to elevate supplier quality performance. It is imperative that suppliers improve their quality standards.

MBNQA CRITERIA

The MBNQA emphasizes seven categories, and its goal is to help organizations focus on quality, customer satisfaction, and so on. The following list presents the items, categories, and point values in their entirety.

Item	Category	Point Value
1.0	Leadership	**90**
1.1	Senior executive leadership	45
1.2	Leadership system and organization	25
1.3	Public responsibility and corporate citizenship	20
2.0	Information and analysis	**75**
2.1	Management of information and data	20
2.2	Competitive comparisons and benchmarking	15
2.3	Analysis and use of company-level data	40
3.0	Strategic planning	**55**
3.1	Strategy development	35
3.2	Strategy deployment	20
4.0	Human resource development and management	**140**
4.1	Human resource planning and evaluation	20
4.2	High-performance work systems	45
4.3	Employee education, training, and development	50
4.4	Employee well-being and satisfaction	25
5.0	Process management	**140**
5.1	Design and introduction of products and services	40

Item	Category	Point Value
5.2	Process management: product and service production and delivery	40
5.3	Process management: support services	30
5.4	Management of supplier performance	30
6.0	**Business results**	**250**
6.1	Product and service quality results	75
6.2	Company operational and financial results	130
6.3	Supplier performance results	45
7.0	**Customer focus and satisfaction**	**250**
7.1	Customer and market knowledge	30
7.2	Customer relationship management	30
7.3	Customer satisfaction determination	30
7.4	Customer satisfaction results	100
7.5	Customer satisfaction comparison	60
TOTAL POINTS		**1000**

As already discussed, the MBNQA is a national quality award focusing on the system of quality for organizations. Therefore, the examiners of the MBNQA look throughout an organization to discover if, in fact, it is quality driven, if quality is documented and—perhaps the most critical characteristic—if the organization's quality efforts are effective. The answers to these concerns are given to the examiners through their book audit as well as their physical audit of the organization.

The specific analysis follows in a condensed format. For an exhaustive discussion on the specificity of each element, see U.S. Department of Commerce (1995) and Heaphy and Gruska (1995).

1.0. *Leadership* (90 points). This category examines senior executives' personal leadership and involvement in creating and sustaining a customer focus, clear values and expectations, and a leadership system that promotes performance excellence. Also examined is how the values and expectations are integrated into the company's management system, including how the company addresses its public responsibilities and corporate citizenship.

2.0. *Information and analysis* (75 points). This category examines the management and effectiveness of the use of data and information to support customer-driven performance excellence and marketplace success.

3.0. *Strategic planning* (55 points). This category examines how the company sets strategic directions and how it determines key plan requirements. Also examined is how the plan requirements are translated into an effective performance management system.

4.0. *Human resource development and management* (140 points). This category examines how the workforce is enabled to develop and use its full potential, aligned with the company's performance objectives. Also examined are the company's efforts to build and maintain an environment conducive to performance excellence, full participation, and personal and organizational growth.

5.0. *Process management* (140 points). This category examines the key aspects of process management, including customer-focused design; product and service delivery processes; support services; and supply management involving all work units, including research and development. Also, this category examines how key processes are designed, effectively managed, and improved to achieve higher performance.

6.0. *Business results* (250 points). This category examines the company's performance and improvement in key business areas—product and service quality, productivity and operational effectiveness, supply quality, and financial performance indicators linked to these areas. Also examined are performance levels relative to competitors.

7.0. *Customer focus and satisfaction* (250 points). This category examines the company's systems for customer learning and for building and maintaining customer relationships. Also examined are levels and trends in key measures of business success—customer satisfaction and retention, market share, and satisfaction relative to competitors.

SCORING SYSTEM

The system for scoring applicant responses to examination items and for developing feedback is based on three evaluation dimensions: approach, deployment, and results.

Approach

Approach refers to how the applicant addresses the item requirements—the methods used. The factors used to evaluate approaches include the following:

- Appropriateness of the methods to the requirements.
- Effectiveness of use of the methods, that is, the degree to which the approach is systematic, integrated, and consistently applied; embodies evaluation and improvement cycles; and is based on information and data that are objective and reliable.
- Evidence of innovation. This includes significant and effective adaptations of approaches used in other applications or types of business.

In real terms, this means that the approach is prevention based and deals with: tools and techniques, integration, and improvement cycles.

Deployment

Deployment refers to the extent to which the applicant's approach is applied to all requirements of the item. The factors used to evaluate deployment include the following:

- Use of the approach in addressing business and item requirements.
- Use of the approach by all appropriate work units.

In real terms, this means that deployment deals with all transactions with customers and suppliers, the public, and so on; operations and processes; and products and services.

Results

Results refers to outcomes in achieving the purposes given in the item. The factors used to evaluate results include the following:

- Current performance levels.
- Performance levels relative to appropriate comparisons and/or benchmarks.
- Rate, breadth, and importance of performance improvements; demonstration of sustained improvement and/or sustained high-level performance.

In real terms, this means that results deal with quality levels, rate of improvement, sustaining improvement, and competitive comparisons.

FUNDAMENTAL PREREQUISITES FOR HEALTHCARE

In the last five years, the healthcare industry, under great pressure from a variety of sources (government, insurance companies, health maintenance organizations, etc.), has looked introspectively at its own operations for improvement. More and more healthcare facilities are drawn to the MBNQA because their management feels that, in conjunction with the principles of TQM, the award provides the essential characteristics for a world-class organization.

The MBNQA process includes the examination criteria and an evaluation process, which provides a tool for planning and improvement. It is not a replacement for the organization's quality improvement or total quality management processes. But it does help organize the various strategies, initiatives, and activities into a framework of TQM to examine the sufficiency of the quality improvement process, to create a common focus throughout the organization, and to identify the strengths and the areas for improvement.

The examination criteria are basically a set of questions covering the scope of total quality management. The seven categories and their examination items provide a framework for organizing the information. The examination items and their areas to address describe the content within the scope of TQM. Most important is the de facto consensus on the scope, framework, and content as defining TQM. The actual examination items are published in the criteria booklet provided by the MBNQA office, and in most cases they are self-explanatory. However, there are many commercial seminars that explain the process, intent, and so on.

Because the MBNQA process is not a replacement for an organization's quality improvement or planning process, it is not another program. Rather, it complements what is already in place from a perspective of total quality management.

So, how does one use the MBNQA? An appropriate use of the information from the MBNQA self-assessment process is to help the organizational planning. Three questions typically are addressed in the traditional planning process:

Where are we now?
Where do we want to be when _____ ?
How are we going to get there?

The implied assumptions usually are not stated. The planned process is assumed to be analytic. Therefore, the answers to the questions are obtained through analysis. The results are task and project oriented, and the process is typically top-down and conducted by a few people in the organization. Usually, the word *we* in the questions is not personal; rather, it is shorthand for *the organization* (certainly not *we the people* in the organization). Planning is designed to produce orderly results, not change. But what results? Planning is inherently divisive, because the plan defines and incorporates the specifics of what will be done and what will not be done. Objective criteria based on organizational requirements must be used in the decisions to avoid creating winners and losers. Planning must be process oriented to ensure that people feel they were given the opportunity to be heard. Consequently, planning must be preceded by direction setting, which is a leadership and decision-making process, not a planning process. Direction setting involves deciding the purpose and mission of the organization, selecting strategies and actions that are required for success, communicating that direction and the rationale, aligning people to the new direction, and building coalitions committed to achieving the vision. The traditional planning process is based on analysis. Leadership is coping with change, which is all about people. The future cannot be planned. Creating the future is a leadership responsibility.

The direction setting and related plans inherently involve change, which will be both personal and cultural. The people who will be making the changes—quite often personal changes—need to be involved in developing the strategic direction and planning the changes required. Clearly, a broader context built on leadership and involving people is required.

Leadership has many unique obligations, including those of having a perspective on the total organization, defining its purpose and mission, developing the fundamental strategies, promoting teamwork, integrating contributions, and communicating. Although all people in the organization can help, these obligations *cannot* be delegated.

An important aspect is defining the character for the organization. Broad participation is beneficial, but the leadership must decide. Questions to be answered include the following:

- What business are we in?
- What services should we provide?
- Who are the potential customers?
- What will distinguish our services from others?
- For what do we want to be known?
- What unmatchable advantages should we try to create?
- What are the key success factors for the organization?
- What unique organizational capability is required?
- What knowledge and skills should be common?
- What strengths should be retained and enhanced?
- What are the areas for improvement?
- What are the organizational goals?
- What are the organizational strategies for achieving the goals?

Certainly, all people should have the opportunity to contribute their ideas and reasons on what the character of the organization should be. A successful definition will likely require an interactive process. Many ideas will be offered. All should be challenged with a consensus evaluation. Leadership must integrate and ultimately decide the answers to the questions needed to create the required focus and must provide the guidance necessary to set the strategic direction.

The strategic direction should be communicated to everyone in the organization in clear, simple language, which is easy to understand and remember. The explanation and reinforcement by actions will create richness in meaning.

Finally, leadership has the obligation to select the method for strategic business management because the strategic direction and related plans are not enough. The method to manage implementation and to constantly reinforce the strategic direction helps explain and give further meaning to the strategic direction through communication by action of what leadership believes to be important. That importance must be built into the management process, with leadership devoting a major amount of time to mentoring the implementation of the strategic direction. For success, decisions must reflect the strategic direction, which inherently gives the decisions a long-term focus—a major challenge in most organizations.

MBNQA APPLICATION PROCESS

This description of the MBNQA process is limited to those key elements required to use the process for improvement. Those key elements are the examination criteria, the self-description, and the self-assessment based on the scoring system with its descriptive scoring guidelines. The annual MBNQA application guidelines and the education and training materials for the board of examiners provide the details. Also, for additional information, see Heaphy and Gruska (1995).

Since the examination criteria are generic and descriptive (as opposed to specific and prescriptive), they apply to all businesses and most organizations, including healthcare and nonprofit organizations. The examination criteria also apply to the internal structure of the organization, although some specific items may not be applicable. The eligibility restrictions required to apply for the award are not restrictions for improvement.

The examination criteria are a set of directions or commands for the application. The scope of the questions encompasses total quality management. The set of questions is organized into seven categories, with each having a number of examination items. The detailed questions in the examination items and the areas that are to be addressed in the examination criteria define the content for TQM. The examination criteria describe the *whats* of TQM. The questions ask for a description of the *hows* used by the organization. Accordingly, the examination criteria provide the scope, content, and framework for organizing a description of total quality of an organization from the perspective of total quality management. (In total, there are 50 areas to address in the guideline.)

The scoring system, which was discussed in an earlier section, is based on three evaluation dimensions of approach, deployment, and results, which further define the content associated with each examination item. The scoring guidelines provide a descriptive scale for numerical evaluation. Overall, the scoring system is prevention based and diagnostic and provides a description of excellence.

All the above factors should be comprehended in the self-assessment. It is of paramount importance that the concepts and principles be well understood as a prerequisite for their use for improvement because the concepts and principles embodied in the examination criteria and scoring system have broad and deep meanings and applications. The need for a consultant and/or appropriate and applicable training should be carefully examined and may be required to avoid compromising the potential benefits.

SUGGESTED EXTENSION OF MBNQA CRITERIA

For purposes of improvement, it may be appropriate to extend the scope of the questions to the total business or organization. Since integration among the categories is also an important aspect of TQM, it may be appropriate to add some explicit questions on interdependence and integration. Also, each organization has unique facets for which specific additional questions may be appropriate.

The obvious extension is from total quality management to total business or total organization. Additional examination items could include strategic direction, financial performance, and other items unique to the organization. A tailored list of items examining the strategic direction should be developed for the specific organization, comprehending the generic leadership obligations described in the section on leadership responsibilities of the criteria booklet provided by the MBNQA office.

Additional examination items and broadened content for the MBNQA examination items could be included to expand the seven categories to a total organizational focus. For example, category 3 (strategic planning) could be expanded to total organizational planning. In this context, information about financial planning, resource planning, and capital planning with an extended set of measurements may be appropriate.

An omission by the MBNQA, but something that could be added to the total organization quality (TOQ) program for improvement, concerns innovation, research, and development. This includes creating products and services that surprise and delight customers. Such products and services create wants, excitement, and their own markets and are not just responses to customer needs and expectations. Another omission by the MBNQA that can be included in the TOQ program is more emphasis on responsiveness or speed of producing quality results. Broader questions on the recognition and reward systems are also appropriate because they must relate to the total organizational process, not just total quality management.

Finally, a separate category on integration should be considered, one that would identify the major interdependencies that are important to the organization. As with the other examination items, approach, deployment, and results are equally or more important for integration. Benchmarks for integration are appropriate, as are trend charts demonstrating improvements in integration. Integration should address the interdependencies among the categories. One description of the interrelationships is shown in Figure 9–1.

Figure 9–1 uses the "right-side-up" organizational model in which customers are placed at the top. Without customers, no organization can exist for long. Leadership is shown at the bottom supporting the entire organizational process. Adjacent categories are highly interdependent. Leadership has a major role in creating the overall plan, which defines the quality assurance (systems and processes); the expected quality results; and the satisfaction systems, processes, and expected results for customer satisfaction.

F I G U R E   9–1

A Model for Integration of MBNQA in Healthcare

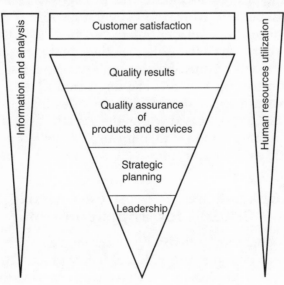

Quality assurance of products and services (systems and processes) produces the quality results, which, in turn, produce the customer satisfaction results. Human resource utilization integrates the activities from leadership to customers as does information and analysis. This is shown as a triangle depicting the integration and summarization of data into information—from the detailed data gathered by the people responsible for individual actions to summaries required by leadership for the management of the total organization.

The examination criteria for improvement should be broader than for the selection of award winners because the diagnostic need is broader. For improvement, the identification of deficiencies is needed now, as are examinations of the sufficiency of organizational strategies and systems. For the award, the omitted content in the examination criteria is explicit only. Success requires that each of these areas be addressed, and, therefore, they are implicitly contained in the MBNQA criteria. For example, without attention to the financial aspects, funds may not be available for research and development or even for training. The diagnostic requirement for improvement dictates that the expanded criteria be explicit so that the evaluation can be made now, rather than just reflected through customer satisfaction results in the long term.

It should be emphasized that the MBNQA has only seven examination categories. However, I suggest an eighth category for integration to show the reader that the intent of the MBNQA does not stop with the seven items. Rather, the intent is to show that integration of whatever the organization says about itself is consistent and effective throughout. The discussion of the eighth category is a recommendation and only provides information about how the MBNQA is diffused within the organization. It is not necessary for an organization to identify an extra category. It will simply be a little easier for all concerned.

Application of Extended MBNQA Criteria for Improvement

The fundamentals, extended MBNQA criteria and the self-assessment, can now be combined with the change process to create, develop, plan, and implement orderly change toward total quality management. A strong leadership role is required for all phases but particularly for creating the definition of the desired future state.

Self-Assessment

The self-assessment is intended to answer the traditional planning question, Where are we now? and to develop the perceived need for further change. The benefits from self-assessment are many. The assessment is conducted by those most knowledgeable, who are in a better position to relate the criteria to the current status. Describing and explaining the current status helps understanding and ownership of the areas identified for improvement. Peer pressure helps to counteract the "good news syndrome." Personal integrity is also enhanced if the self-assessment is completed without distortion. Overall, the self-assessment creates a rapid learning process. The stronger the method of self-assessment, the better the results. The examination criteria, developed independently through a consensus process, define the scope and content of questions which may surface during the difficult issues. Team processes facilitate more discussion and understanding and help ensure objectivity for describing the current status.

The assessment teams should be carefully crafted. Team champions for each of the categories should be selected from senior management. A network of members from the departments and facilities (if appropriate) should be assigned to each champion to form a team for each category. Members from senior managers should be assigned to the champions to form the team for category 1—leadership. A team of team champions should have the responsibility for category 8—integration. The team relationships should not be hierarchical. Team processes should be used for self-assessment (self-description and self-evaluation). Again, a knowledgeable consultant should be considered to facilitate the self-assessment. A major role of the consultant is to question claims to ensure that they are clearly supported.

Documentation of both the self-assessment and the evaluation is required. The mindset that "we all know the current state and therefore have no need for documentation" must be avoided, as should the opposite tendency to document everything. The limit to about 75 pages required in the MBNQA application forces simplification, which should be based on better understanding and not deletions. Understanding typically requires the sequence of adding more and more data and detail as part of the identification of the underlying principles and trends, which then leads to better understanding and to simplification. Documentation should be sufficient to effectively communicate with others to understand the interdependencies and integration. A minimum level of documentation to begin the self-description process is a list of key points describing approach, deployment, and results together with trend charts for the results.

The evaluation process should also be documented, perhaps on pages opposite to the self-assessment. Strengths, areas for improvement, and questions for further study should be identified. Team processes should be used to provide a broad perspective and help ensure objectivity. The generic and descriptive scoring criteria in the scoring system also help. A qualified consultant can bring a broad TQM focus and expertise for the evaluation.

The same method of self-assessment should be used for integration and other extensions of the MBNQA examination criteria. To describe and evaluate integration, the approach, deployment, and results must all be considered with insistence on a method for measurement and evidence that the claimed level of integration actually exists. For more information on self-assessment, see Stamatis (1995).

Shared Vision (Desired Future State)

The MBNQA examination criteria with the extended examination items may also be used to organize the definition of the shared vision or desired future state. This definition should describe what the leadership and people in the organization want the organization to be in the long term. The description should include the approach, deployment, and expected results for each examination item. The same team processes should be used to define the desired future state with more emphasis on interdependencies. Recommendations should be solicited from multiple sources for each examination item.

The leadership role is even more important in defining the desired future. There must be a clear definition of goals. Refinement of the organizational definition is required to provide broad guidance for others to use in the definitions of their areas of responsibility. Specifically, drafts of categories 1 (leadership) and 8 (integration) together with the broad goals for the organization, approved by leadership, are required to define that broad guidance. The completion of the definition of the desired future state by the teams and others is an interactive, synergistic, integrative process. Changes to all of the categories, including those developed by leadership, will be required to incorporate the many good ideas and to develop consistency.

The definition of the desired future state must be much more than just responding to areas for improvement identified in the self-assessment. Response to the identified opportunities is important, but it is reactive. The leadership and people in the organization must also be proactive by creating and redesigning the organizational definition, answering questions described in the section on leadership responsibilities, integrating the many good ideas from the teams and others, and communicating the vision for the organization. Leadership and redesign of the strategies, systems, and processes are also required to create a high-performance organization. The organizational capability as defined by the principal systems and processes must be clearly described and evaluated for sufficiency. Another perspective on the importance of the shared vision is provided by considering what is likely to happen without one. Each person will likely have a different vision with some elements in common, but not all. Decisions on short-term plans will be made individually from the different visions and will often be reactive in response to short-term considerations and self-interests. Coordination will be difficult, and progress will be slow. Of course, this is where documentation is absolutely required, along with much dialogue to ensure understanding. However, the tendency to be too detailed must be resisted.

An evaluation of the description of the desired future state should be made using the same evaluation process. As before, strengths, areas for improvement, and questions should be identified and documented. The definition of the character of the organization and the goals should be used to assess the importance of the strengths and areas for improvement. It is not necessary for the organization to do everything. But it must be strong in the areas critical to the organizational definition, character, and goals.

Integration and consistency require special attention. Because of interdependence among the categories and among the departments and facilities (if appropriate) within an organization, all must have the same understanding of the desired future state and their roles and responsibilities in creating complementary elements of that future state. The description of methods for development and maintaining integration should also be described and evaluated for approach, deployment, and expected results.

The description of the desired future state is not complete without an evaluation of sufficiency. Are the planned changes implementable and capable of producing the expected results? This requires a critical examination of the effectiveness of the approaches. Leadership and the teams should insist on persuasive explanations and arguments. It is not sufficient to rely on the old way of doing things. Carefully study the areas for improvement in the self-assessment of the current state to ensure that the important opportunities are addressed. Do not try to be everything to everybody. Use the organizational definition, character, and goals as the decision criteria for sufficiency.

The definition of the desired future state is a continuous process, which should be refined and updated periodically. A broad focus should be maintained to reflect the long-term perspective and to provide flexibility to adapt to a changing environment. The detail should be in the plans describing the good next steps, which should have a short-term focus.

Example of Education and Training   To clarify the description of the current and desired future states and their uses, consider the following example for education and training (E&T). The example is a hypothetical examination item stating: Describe the process for identifying, developing, delivering, and improving the education and training. The description should obviously address approach, deployment, and results.

Current State   The key organization for E&T is the training committee. This committee is composed of representatives from all of the departments, and its responsibility is to identify the courses required, set the priorities for development, guide the development, and review the course evaluation results. The courses are developed by the E&T Department with assistance from experts on various subjects from both inside and outside the organization. Courses are offered on a regular basis with the individual divisions, and departments and plants have responsibility for scheduling their people to the various courses. An evaluation of the course and of the instructor is made by participants at the end of each course.

Desired Future State   The purpose of the E&T is to provide education and training services in support of organizational goals. Accordingly, the E&T requirements are identified internally with the planning process. Developed by the departments, each job description includes a listing of the knowledge and skills required. General knowledge and skills are also described for each department. Course improvements are identified continually and formally during the planning process.

The E&T Department facilitates course development. Externally available standardized courses are used whenever possible. Subject-matter experts, consultants, and others participate in the development of specialized courses. Most courses have different modules for managers, supervisors, and willing workers. Regardless of what courses are chosen for training, it is of paramount importance that their design is based on adult E&T principles. Course schedules are developed based on organizational plans to meet the needs of the departments, which have the overall responsibility for educating and training their people. The delivery process is interactive with the supervisor of the participant.

Advance notice is sent to the participant and supervisor to prepare for the course. This notice includes the purpose, expectations, selection of project for application, and arrangements for handling the participant's work during his or her absence. This minimizes the interruptions during the formal part of the E&T.

The class and workshop work is immediately followed by a dialogue with the supervisor discussing what was learned, how it can be used, application to a specific project to reinforce the learning, and the required guidance and support. Several months after the formal course, a student evaluation of the entire delivery process is made and communicated confidentially to the E&T Department.

The process has been deployed throughout the organization and the survey results indicate a high degree of involvement by supervisors in the E&T process.

Observations   There are many significant observations from the two descriptions of the organization described in this hypothetical E&T examination item.

- The description of the current state is incomplete. Deployment and results on the effectiveness of the approach are inadequately described.
- More words are needed to describe the desired future state. The expanded description communicates an image that people should be able to visualize and want to be a part of. Note that, over time, the description can be shortened and simplified as broader understanding develops and the image of the future state is taken for granted.
- Many organizations are involved in the successful use of E&T, requiring other departments and supervisors to take on additional roles. For example, supervisors learn first and arrange for work replacement during their employees' classwork. Also, immediate application is part of E&T for the participant, and the subject-matter experts assist in the development of the course material.
- The evaluation determines the effectiveness of the entire process, including the effectiveness of the participating departments and supervisors.
- The description of the future state is also incomplete.

Most of these observations relate to the interdependencies required for successful use of adult E&T. Plans must be developed simultaneously with team processes.

Good Next Steps and Resistance to Change

The good next steps and the actions to reduce the resistance to change should be planned together. This part of the plan is focused on the short term to define some of the immediate actions to move toward the description of the desired future state and to establish the long-term direction. Typically, this part describes the first year or two of the organizational plan and requires funding of the projects. A macro description and time frame of the overall transitional plan to the desired future state is needed to help in the selection of the most important changes to implement in the current year. Furthermore, broad guidance providing an overall definition of the good next steps and the actions to reduce the resistance to change is required from the leadership. This guidance is a prerequisite for development of consistent plans by the departments and functional units within the total organization.

For a successful change process the responsibility for each change must be clearly defined and assigned to the appropriate personnel. Furthermore, it must meet the needs of the total organization. The processes for defining the good next steps for all of the individual examination items should be highly interactive, to ensure that the many individual changes are aligned and consistent. The detail should include the areas for improvement. The individual actions should be selected based on the context of the desired future state and organizational goals. In this process, the boss is the description of the desired future state and organizational goals, which should provide the unity of purpose for the team efforts. Again, note the need for imagery in the descriptions. With good imagery, people can visualize the future and want to be a part of that future. The development of the interdependencies requires special attention. Unless the interdependencies are appropriately comprehended in the plan, the implementation will bring to the surface omissions, misunderstandings, and conflicts, which will compromise the overall implementation. Interdependent changes will be required to address the omissions, disconnects, and conflicts, which at best will slow down the implementation.

This is another example of the importance of integration, which is a primary leadership responsibility, and of the need for a new category—perhaps integration with a well-defined set of examination items. But integration is also the responsibility of each person to address. Organizationally, this requires working on issues that are "horizontal and outward" (participation and commitment) in addition to the "inward and vertical" (authority and control). Although each person has a responsibility for the horizontal and outward aspects, the majority responsibility belongs to supervisors, managers, and executives. Consistency is required for the short term (good next steps) and the long term (desired future state).

A few final thoughts on the resistance to change. Communication and participation are important elements. The future state should be described with sufficient imagery so that people want to create that future and understand what their roles and responsibilities are in creating that future. Explain why, not just what is required, so that everyone understands which actions are required and why they are important. The explanations will become the basis for many future decisions required for implementation and improvement. Use the "circular" model of retraining the old practices and systems until the new ones are fully implemented and working as intended (Stamatis 1995). Create a learning environment. Require as much or more justification not to change as to change. Help people become comfortable with change as the norm. Establish a team environment with the appropriate employees to provide clear expectations for addressing the many interdependencies.

REFERENCES

Heaphy, M. S., and G. F. Gruska. *The Malcolm Baldrige National Quality Award.* Reading, Mass.: Addison-Wesley, 1995.

Nordeen, D. L. "An Opportunity to Improve Total Quality Management: The National Quality Award." In *Quality Concepts 1991: A National Forum on Total Quality Management* (conference proceedings). Detroit: Engineering Society, 1991, pp. 403–23.

Stamatis, D. H. *Total Quality Service.* Delray Beach, Fla.: St. Lucie Press, 1995.

U.S. Department of Commerce. *Malcolm Baldrige National Quality Award 1995 Award Criteria.* Gaithersburg, Md.: U.S. Department of Commerce, Technology Administration, National Institute of Standards and Technology, 1995.

CHAPTER 10

Marketing System Design

Most marketers have been exposed to the saying, "A better mousetrap will not necessarily result in the customers beating a path to your door." How, then, does one market a service such as healthcare? This chapter will discuss the process of developing a healthcare service marketing system. This discussion is included because I believe that the process of marketing in healthcare is essential to the overall success of the organization.

A SYSTEM FOR SERVICE MARKETING DEVELOPMENT

For the marketing system to be effective, its impact on the overall program must be considered. Market feasibility information must be established before the development of such a system is undertaken. The development of marketing feasibility information includes the analysis of the service, the potential (target) population, and the resources available for marketing that service. Specific tools in analyzing these items may be focus groups, benchmarking, quality function deployment, surveys, and so on. For details on these tools and their application, see Camp (1995); Stamatis (1995a); Akao (1990); and Berwick, Godfrey, and Roessner (1990). Each of these analyses may occur concurrently or, if performed by a team, may be in sequence. The results from each analysis are used to build the marketing program system, which in turn is used to arrive at a realistic perspective in conjunction with other information. This chain of information, finally, provides the foundation for decision making and planning complete service analysis (Figures 10–1 and 10–2).

COMPLETE SERVICE ANALYSIS

A complete service analysis is a thorough, systematic, and factual statement of the attributes of the service. From simple clear statements of the service characteristics through the service advantages, this analysis seeks to distinguish your organization's service from someone else's. That is, it tries to position the service within the competition or outside the competition as a leader for that service.

Once the attributes of the service have been defined, then a relational analysis takes place. The function of this analysis is to compare the same or similar services with other providers of that service. It is imperative when this analysis takes place that the comparison takes a nondefensive, noncontroversial form and remains simple and concise.

The advantages of the proposed or existing service must all be stated, in order to move to the next point of concern, which is to state the obstacles from the competition or your own organization. Obstacles are those considerations or activities that cause a potential customer to decide *not* to purchase or use the specific service. It is critical to concisely state each possible obstacle.

Having stated all possible obstacles, the analysis moves to state the uses of the product. These uses may consider specific applications as well as general or overall use. This phase seeks to state all possible uses of the service—conventional and creative. The generated list of such an activity should be as extensive as possible. A reminder at this point! It is of extreme importance to consider all possible applications and opportunities that have been stated from different points of view, until everyone is comfortable with the outcome.

The listing of the service uses may then be used for the next phase, which is to state the end results or expectations of the service use. This considers the results and ramifications which

F I G U R E   10–1

System for Service Marketing Development

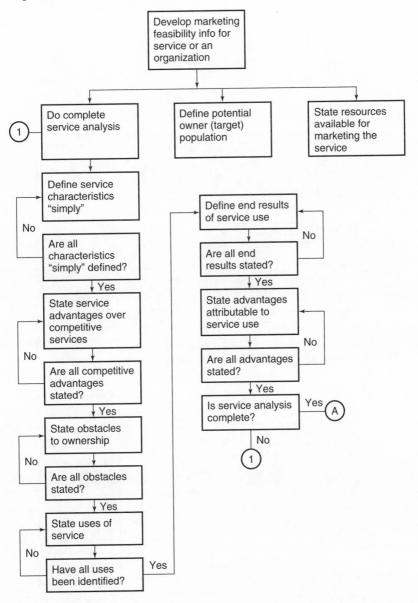

F I G U R E   10–1   (continued)

System for Service Marketing Development

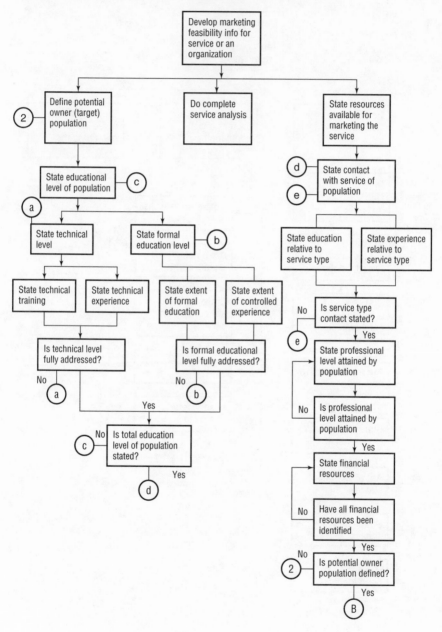

F I G U R E   10–2

Design of Marketing Service Feasibility and System

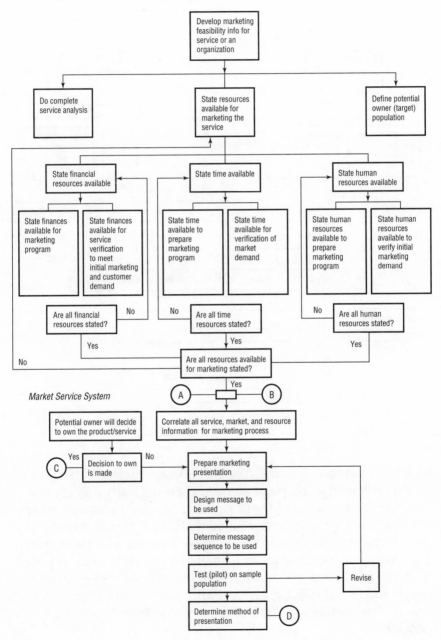

F I G U R E   10–2   (continued)

Design of Marketing Service Feasibility and System

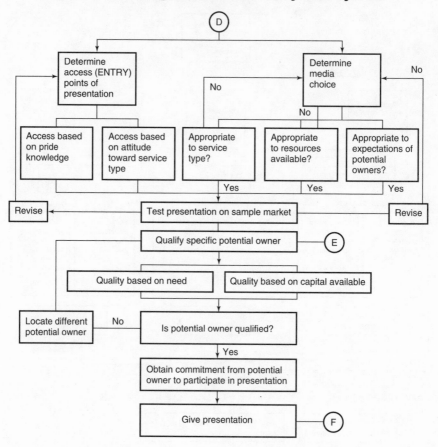

will be marketed or are currently being marketed from the user's perspective and point of view. Having clearly and concisely stated every known end result possible, the final phase of stating the utility of using the service is to make sure that differentiation exists between other services that are similar or the same. Remember! We want the customer to purchase our service as opposed to someone else's. In this endeavor, one may even use the failure mode and effect analysis (FMEA) for a more effective resolution. For a detailed explanation of the FMEA, see Stamatis (1995b).

F I G U R E   10–2   (continued)

Design of Marketing Service Feasibility and System

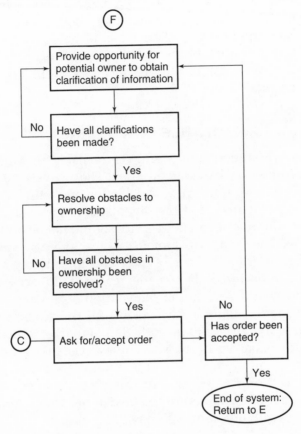

DEFINITION OF TARGET POPULATION

Whereas the educational level would be an important demographic characteristic to address from a product orientation and for many services, in the healthcare service orientation, educational level does not generally play a major role. What does play a role, however, is the financial status and resources of the potential user population. Depending on the mission of the organization, this definition of the target population may make or break the success of the organization.

Note that I have refrained from identifying the customer and the target population as strictly "the patient." As already mentioned, in healthcare there are many customers with their own needs, wants, and expectations. As a consequence, when the organization is ready to define the marketing strategy, the appropriate and applicable customer has to be defined separately. Also, I have refrained from identifying the organization as a "hospital." Obviously, healthcare includes more organizations than just hospitals.

RESOURCES AVAILABLE FOR MARKETING

Realistic consideration of the resources available for marketing the service is critical to the overall program. The analysis must be careful in stating those resources available for marketing a particular service. Any resources that the organization has available which are not used for marketing this service should not be considered in the analysis. The resources of finances, time, and personnel should be considered seriously. Each of these considers two points of the application of resources. First, is the resource (finances, time, personnel) available to use in the preparation of the marketing program? Second, is the resource available for the design and implementation of the service to meet the initial market demand? After an exhaustive analysis of these two questions, the organization is ready to make a statement about the resources available. If there is more information needed or something has changed, then additions and/or modifications are accepted as necessary. At this point, the market feasibility information is complete.

MARKETING PROGRAM SYSTEM

The marketing program system has seven basic elements (Figure 10–2).

   1. The first element is the statement of the precise objective. Normally, for a marketing system, the objective is that the potential customer will decide to use the service. If the potential customer does decide to use the service, the system moves to the last element, accepting the service. If the potential customer does not make the positive "ownership" decision, the system continues to the second element.

2. Preparation of a marketing presentation is undertaken with the support and information attained in the marketing feasibility information analysis. All of this information is available for the preparer in making decisions for the marketing program presentation. Preparing the presentation includes designing the messages to be used and determining the sequence of the messages. This should be done with full awareness of the target audience of the presentation. The target market's educational level, professional level, and previous contact with the service, for example, all have an impact on presentation decisions. The messages should be systematically designed to alter the audience's basic information and attitudes and motivate the audience to take action (purchase or receive the service). Having designed the messages and sequenced them, they should be tested on a sample population and revised as necessary to achieve the desired response.

3. Next, consider the method of presentation. The media choice must be made based on the appropriateness of the media to the service type, the resources of the organization available for media, and the expectations of the potential target population. For example, if the presentation will normally be made on a one-to-one basis, then a five-projector, multimedia slide presentation may not be as appropriate as a short movie or videotape, which could easily be shown on portable equipment, requiring little setup time. Similarly, use of a flip chart may not go far when addressing larger groups of potential users or decision makers. The other consideration to be made in the method of presentation is the points of entry. If a potential customer has had experience with a genetic service but not the particular service being marketed, there should be one or more access points available during the presentation to consider individuals with different needs for information. The person who has had favorable technical experience with the trial type but needs more end-result information to make a positive decision to use the service should be able to enter the presentation at the most constructive point.

4. After deciding on the method of presentation, test the presentation on a sample population. Revise it as appropriate and then retest it.

5. The next element of the marketing program system is the qualification of the potential user. The potential user (person or organization) must be qualified based on need of the service and on the capital available to support a decision to use the service. If either consideration is not met, the potential user is not qualified, and another potential user should be sought and asked to commit to the program.

6. The marketing presentation is then given. The potential user is given the opportunity (during or after the presentation) to clarify information, such as application of the service, end results possible, capital needed, and advantages. After all clarifications have been made, obstacles to ownership are dealt with and resolved individually (obstacle by obstacle).

7. After all obstacles to ownership have been resolved, the potential customer is asked for the order, which is accepted. Should the order not be given, the system is reentered at the point where obstacles to ownership are resolved, and followed through again. If the order is given, it is accepted, and the system is reentered at the point a qualified potential owner is being sought, and followed through to completion.

MARKET SEGMENTATION

When developing corporate or marketing strategy, it is important to identify the different market segments that make up the total market. A market segment is a group of customers with similar or related buying motives. The members of the segment have similar needs, wants, and expectations. A focus on market segments allows a company to tailor its products, services, pricing, distribution, and communication message to meet the specific needs of a market.

The opposite of market segmentation is mass marketing. Segmentation allows a smaller organization to successfully attack a larger one by concentrating resources at the specific point of competition. Any market can be segmented. The radiology market, for example, can be segmented into the x-ray market, ultrasound market, computed tomography (CAT scan) market, and so on.

To segment a market, you need to know who the customers are, what they buy, how they buy, when they buy, why they buy, and where they buy. In healthcare, segmentation seems to be the future. There are now hospital service lines or entire healthcare facilities that specialize in specific clinical services, such as trauma management, coronary care, pediatrics, and heart surgery. These services aim to better meet the needs, wants, and expectations of the customer.

R E F E R E N C E S

Akao, Y., ed. *Quality Function Deployment,* trans. Mazur, G. H. Cambridge, Mass.: Productivity Press, 1990.

Berwick, D. M.; A. B. Godfrey; and J. Roessner. *Curing Health Care.* San Francisco: Jossey-Bass, 1990.

Camp, R. *Benchmarking.* Milwaukee: Quality Press, 1995.

Stamatis, D. H. *Total Quality Service.* Delray Beach, Fla.: St. Lucie Press, 1995a.

———. *Failure Mode and Effect Analysis: FMEA from Theory to Execution.* Milwaukee: Quality Press, 1995b.

PART TWO

Deployment of TQM

Breakthrough Strategy and Implementation

CHAPTER 11

How to Implement Total Quality Management

This chapter describes the implementation strategy for TQM. The discussion focuses on a seven-step approach, which identifies the minimum requirements for successful implementation. For a lengthy discussion of implementing TQM, the reader is encouraged to read Stamatis (1991, 1995), Scherkenback (1988), and Griffiths (1990).

As already discussed, TQM is a philosophy that an organization may use to define its quality level and to achieve world-class recognition through new standards of excellence. To implement this philosophy, an organization must understand at least two concepts: (1) variability and (2) process. Furthermore, it must be willing to reduce this variability by using processes that are broken down into small, simple tasks, parts, and so on, which can be routinely managed. How do we do this? By implementing TQM through seven steps (Table 11–1).

IMPLEMENTATION STEPS

Step 1: Energize the Organization with Quality Awareness

It is management's responsibility to announce systematically the changes that are about to take place in the organization. It is imperative at this first step to define the role of quality and what is

TABLE 11-1

Seven Steps for TQM Implementation

Foundation	Energize the organization with quality awareness
	Change the culture of the organization
Building blocks	Define the scope of your commitment to the organization as a whole
	Identify key process and product or service variables
	Implement statistical process control (SPC)
	Incorporate process improvement activities in the organization
Feedback/evaluation	Assess the quality improvement in the organization

the organization's expectations of quality. This may be transmitted with meetings, slogans, missions, values, and so on.

Step 2: Change the Culture of the Organization

This second step is more than the initial training of the workforce in classic statistical process control (SPC) and how statistics may be used effectively in managing and understanding the business within the overall TQM discipline. It is more than training in problem-solving techniques and team philosophy. It is about creating a positive environment to make the surroundings such that everywhere employees look, the things they hear, the feeling they get all day, must reflect quality and a customer focus. This step must also address the process required to make people change. The training for successful TQM implementation in this step must be done with the following in mind:

- *Vision*—must be logical.
- *Current snapshot*—must be feasible.
- *Commitment*—must be capable.
- *Selling*—must be desirable.
- *Habit building*—must be full in applicable positive evidence, creating a positive reinforcement.

Creating a positive environment is about nurturing change in people. As a consequence, all training must focus on the following: building trust; reducing fear of the unknown; creating concern for quality through personal ownership and empowerment; providing positive communication; breaking down interdepartmental and intradepartmental barriers; uncovering (positively without fear) problems, issues, and concerns; being open-minded; soliciting, rather than waiting for, input; providing timely feedback; treating your employees with personal and professional respect; soliciting (actively) ways of improving quality; fostering employee initiative, ingenuity, and creativity; and empowering employees with true authority and responsibility for their own work environment.

Finally, if the destination is logical, if the path is feasible, if the workers view themselves as capable, and the end result is desirable, there are few limits to implementing TQM.

Step 3: Define the Scope of Your Commitment to the Organization as a Whole

To define the scope of your commitment to the organization as a whole is one of the most difficult steps in TQM implementation. Some of the considerations toward these definitions are the following:

- *Customer orientation.* Satisfying internal and external customers by meeting their needs, wants, and expectations is the primary consideration.

- *Quality goals.* Many U.S. companies are embracing "six sigma" as a business strategy to increase quality. Others are jumping on the bandwagon of ISO 9000 certification. Still others are committed to the Malcolm Baldrige National Quality Award criteria.

In the healthcare industry this requires designs that accommodate reasonable variation in service processes that yield consistently uniform results. The key to a process definition lies in the ability to identify the steps involved so that they can be individually measured and analyzed. The process definition helps validate and sets standards for what service the customer wants and which services are required to adequately support it.

Step 4: Identify Key Process and Product or Service Variables

In this step we are ready to measure and analyze the process or processes that we defined in the previous step. Our goal here is to provide a plan for the following:

- *Definition.* Definitions help us measure the output. Therefore, do we really have the appropriate definitions for our processes?
- *Evaluation.* We gather and study information about the process and service variables. Therefore, have we identified the appropriate and applicable tools and methods for a worthwhile evaluation?
- *Validation.* Validate the information gathered from the evaluation step with the requirements of the customer. Therefore, do we have an effective way of validating our evaluation results?
- *Organization.* Once the valid list of requirements for our quality has been identified, we can develop, organize, and systematize the plan.

A typical plan may include:

- *Quality mission/objective/policy.* Have we really internalized the concept and ramifications of the quality mission, objective, or policy of the organization? Are they effective? Are they appropriate? Are they real?
- *Description of process.* Do we understand the process? Is there a process flow diagram available?
- *Customer-focused requirements* (if applicable). Do we really provide what the customers want? How can we be sure that they are more than satisfied, that they are delighted?
- *Training and education.* Are special training and educational requirements needed? How do they affect the result or results of this process? Are special certifications required for the operating of the process?
- *Control systems.* How do we measure the effectiveness of this process? How do we know if the results are acceptable?

- *Schedules.* Are specific schedules and sequences unique to this process? How do they affect the results?
- *Action item lists.* What are the items in this process on which we can take action?

It is important to note that in this step a high level of interaction must take place between management and operators. In fact, a critical input of the definition must come from employees close to the task, since they are the ones with the most knowledge regarding the particular task.

Step 5: Implement Statistical Process Control

SPC monitors processes and provides timely information for making quality improvements. It measures the quality performance of people, machines, materials, methods, measurements, and environments. The specific quality tools were addressed in Chapter 6. What is important to note is the position of SPC in the successful implementation stage. Many organizations, especially service industries, claim that they have tried SPC but that it did not work. The reason it does not work in any organization is because steps 2 through 4 have been bypassed. These organizations think that by having an "awareness day" or a plain mission statement, the culture of the organization will change. Unless the commitment of top management is demonstrated over and over again and unless the process and its key characteristics have been defined, SPC will not work. (You may have a statistical process display [SPD] but not a truly SPC program.) That is not a good reason to say that SPC is not applicable. It just means that the organization prematurely tried to implement a tool for improvement. To have an effective SPC program demands hard work and true commitment from everyone.

Key characteristics are defined as those that are fundamental to the design of the process. Without them, the design will not be effective. The key characteristics are formulated by one or more of the following:

- Customer.
- Management (engineering).
- Industry standards.

- Governmental regulations (certification bodies).
- Courts (through malpractice suits).

Eventually the key characteristics will become the key process variables as part of the process. They have to be monitored so that variation can be controlled and minimized.

Step 6: Incorporate Process Improvement Activities in the Organization

The theme of this step is continuous improvement, and that means a direction to excellence for total quality. In real terms of application, it includes:

- A strong customer orientation by everyone.
- Participation by everyone with the common goal of improvement.
- Training for everyone to understand, support, and contribute to total quality.
- Motivation by everyone to achieve total quality through trust, respect, and recognition.
- Services that meet the needs, wants, and expectations of the customer and that delight the customer.
- Information available to everyone in such a way that, by integrating it to products and services, improvement will occur.
- A view of suppliers as partners who are recognized based on their potential and actual value contributing to meeting the requirements for total quality. An interesting approach to inform the customer of this partnership is discussed by Fiorentino (1991).
- A quality culture developed by management in an established value system to reflect total quality in the entire organization.
- Planning total quality in both strategic and financial business objectives.
- Communication encouraged in a two-way approach from bottom-top and top-bottom orientations.
- Effective use of accountability measures for total quality to improve the total system of the organization.

Although all the above points will contribute to improvement, one must realize the way we may tap into that improvement is not really that easy. Some ways to meet new and different challenges quickly and successfully are:

1. Keep raising the standards. Even though we are more aware of quality issues than at any time in our history, low standards are literally killing all sorts of businesses. By raising the standards, a business stands out from the crowd. We must view all standards as the minimum acceptance of quality. An analogy may clarify this point. Think of the professional golfer. If the pro is to continue as a golfer, he or she must *on a continual basis* beat the par of the golf course. If the golfer is as good as par, he or she will not make it to the golf tours. You see, the par is a standard, but it is not good enough if one desires to be a professional golfer.

2. Be prepared to climb the next mountain. We in the American business world are suffering from self-imposed artificial limits, and we are paying the price for it. It is time to reevaluate ourselves. Think of a turtle. For it to take a single step, it must stick its neck out. We must regain the entrepreneurial spirit, and we must begin to take calculated risks without the fear of retaliation, name calling, or discipline of some kind.

3. Keep our eyes off the competition. What the Joneses are doing may not be in our best interest. We must shake off the corporate inferiority complex and move on to develop our own niches of quality, specifications, price, and the like.

4. Defy conventional wisdom. Be ready to move on to uncharted waters on behalf of the customer. It is easy to claim that you are an exceptional captain in the harbor. Your superiority, though, will shine as you handle the ship in the rough open seas.

5. Stay on track. If you know your business and your business culture, your strength becomes knowledge. Do not compromise it. Do it over and over again, until improvements are made.

6. Check your assumptions. Just because it worked yesterday, it may not work today. Because things change, you must review and in some cases challenge your assumptions. After all, remember that assumptions distort and limit the way we think about fundamental issues. Examples are: "Of course, we know the customer," "We are the leaders in our field," "We are the best in our business," "Price is the only thing our customers care about," and "Quality is a waste of time."

7. Be open about what you do. What draws a prospect to do

business with you today is your knowledge and expertise. The only way to communicate the real strengths of your organization is to share your knowledge and experience.

Step 7: Assess the Quality Improvement in the Organization

The theme here is "How do you know?" To answer this question, we must use some statistical methods, qualitative and quantitative, descriptive and inferential, as appropriate and applicable. However, this is only one aspect of total quality. Another aspect is to get more statistically minded workers, scientists, physicians, nurses, and administrators, not only to employ a lot of statisticians.

The fact remains, however, that to do an assessment, we must have an analytic process that transforms raw data into relevant, accurate, timely, and usable strategic knowledge in short time frames. It may be information about the driving force within the marketplace. It may be information about specific services, technologies, and processes. Continuous monitoring and benchmarking of competitors, customers, suppliers, and other forces should be an integral part of the overall strategic management function of all organizations. Continuous monitoring prevents a company from being surprised. By keeping apprised of your process and industry developments, an organization can take appropriate and timely action.

REFERENCES

Fiorentino, P. "Supplier-Day Helps Forge Customer-Supplier Partnership." *Quality Progress*, May 1991, p. 176.

Griffiths, D. N. *Implementing Quality with a Customer Focus.* Milwaukee: Quality Press, 1990.

Scherkenback, W. W. *The Deming Route to Quality and Productivity.* Washington, D. C.: Creep Press Books, 1988.

Stamatis, D. H. "Total Quality Implementation." In *Quality Concepts 1991.* Detroit: Detroit Engineering Society, 1991.

————. *Total Quality Service.* Delray Beach, Fla.: St. Lucie Press, 1995.

CHAPTER 12

Breakthrough Process

This chapter will offer an approach to implement the TQM philosophy and demonstrate the practical application of TQM throughout the healthcare organization. Our basis for understanding and implementing the concepts is based on Dr. W. Edwards Deming's Plan-Do-Check-Act (PDCA) model. We begin as the decision has just been made by the senior management to embark on TQM.

ROLES IN THE ORGANIZATION

To implement the TQM philosophy with breakthrough processes in the entire organization, some organizational requirements must be met. The requirements have to do with the structure of the organization and the persons involved in the implementation of the program. It is beyond the scope of this book to discuss the changing culture of the organization as it involves reengineering. On the other hand, the important persons who will be the main players in the process of implementation are the president (provides the quality leadership), quality council (all senior executives), quality officer, sponsor, facilitator, project (team) leader, task leader, team member, and quality consultant (either internal or external). Not every organization must have these job positions to implement a TQM program; however, these positions are most commonly found in the healthcare industry. Some of the specific roles of these persons follow.

Role of the Quality Council

As members of the quality council, senior executives establish quality direction and goals and provide resources up front. As they review the progress of improvement teams and the quality process, they recognize employees for their efforts and acknowledge employees' apprehensions about change. Quality council members also revise reward systems to incorporate quality improvement efforts as well as participate in quality improvement team presentations and comment on recommended actions. Finally, they attend training courses as participants and serve on quality teams.

Role of the Quality Officer

The quality officer is a senior officer of the organization who is responsible for directing the quality process. This individual serves as a coach, trainer, and resource. The quality officer's role is to:

- Develop quality training plans and capture overall company training requirements.
- Provide structured training to problem improvement teams throughout their existence, including the use of advanced diagnostic tools.
- Monitor improvement team progress and output and provide guidance and feedback.
- Present interim reports to the quality council.
- Act as a communication link to the quality council, maintaining records and evidence of decisions made and implementing agreed-on actions.
- Coordinate the development of a means to capture customer satisfaction on an ongoing basis.
- Ensure that benchmarking occurs—the continuous process of measuring our products and services against our toughest competition and/or the best companies

recognized as world leaders in the products and services we provide.

Role of a Sponsor

A sponsor must be a senior officer. This individual acts as a quality champion. The sponsor supports the project idea and is willing to accept ownership by fostering the improvement team's formation. He or she provides the improvement team with resources to get the job done and guidance and direction if necessary. Finally, the sponsor reassigns job priorities to accommodate team requirements and allocates budgeted funds.

Role of the Facilitator

Perhaps the most important task that the continuous improvement process has to offer in any environment, especially in healthcare, is the role of the facilitator. The facilitator is the navigator, pilot, and engineer of the process. The responsibilities are many. However, four are of paramount importance. They are:

Facilitator Role	Facilitator Actions
Counselor to team leader	Support team leader as much as possible
	Advise on data collection, team dynamics, and obstacles to change
	Help write agenda for team meetings
Cheerleader to team	Actively participate in team meeting as needed
	Advise team on how to overcome obstacles
	Keep team focused on the goal
Teacher of team	Instruct on when and how to use analytic tools
	Ensure changes in process and procedures are documented
	Help institutionalize successful innovations
Advisor to sponsor and management	Ensure ongoing dialogue with team
	Encourage necessary support and feedback to teams
	Help manage the team process
	Help plan expansion strategy and larger change opportunities
	Support other continuous improvement initiatives

Role of the Project Leader

The project, or team, leader acts as a full-fledged team member but also does the following:

- Serves as the contact point for communication on the project status by being the initial contact to the team members' supervisor, keeping the quality officer and team sponsor informed of the team's progress and problems, and seeking support from the team facilitator when needed.
- Maintains official records and evidence of team actions.
- Retains functional authority to implement relevant recommendations after the quality council review.
- Leads problem-solving efforts using project management tools and schedules team activities.

Role of the Task Leader

The task leader serves as the contact point for communication to the team and to subgroup members on their assigned task and is held accountable for accomplishing the assigned task. This individual maintains task records for the project leader and is responsible for scheduling subgroup team activities.

Role of the Team Member

During team development, team members share in a leadership role to help develop a sense of teamwork. They also help define the team's mission statement (also called a problem statement or opportunity statement). A mission statement is unique to each team. The team develops its mission statement after assignment of a problem by the quality improvement council. This responsibility includes identification of the problem, preparation of a problem statement describing the problem or opportunity, and ultimately resolution of that problem statement.

Additionally, each team member:

- Analyzes the symptoms and searches for or theorizes as to the root causes of the problem.
- After verifying that the findings have included all potential causes, agrees on what are considered to be the root causes of the problem.
- Addresses the problem by generating creative and feasible corrective actions.
- Tests theories as to causes, stimulates remedies, and performs test pilots of the remedies.
- Presents recommended corrective actions and solutions while establishing controls to prevent the problem from recurring.
- Implements the solutions using an action plan as a guide.
- Monitors the results of the actions and evaluates the solution.
- Monitors the ongoing process for compliance with intended results.

Finally, all team members should feel personally accountable for the problem's resolution.

Role of the Quality Consultant

The consultant may be internal or external. More than one consultant may be used. The consultant provides training in special topics and projects. This individual also provides special resources as needed.

In addition to the roles just described, specific checklists should be developed to facilitate planning (Table 12–1) and implementation (Tables 12–2 and 12–3).

IMPLEMENTATION PROCESS

At this stage, the process of the breakthrough strategy is ready to be implemented. The process is a four-step approach. The steps are (1) do preliminary work, (2) introduce the concept of continuous

T A B L E   12–1

Checklist for Collecting Data, Experimenting with New Ideas, and Addressing Barriers

With Team Leader and Team
1. Verify analysis
    a. Is team collecting the right data?
    b. Is the method of collection correct and consistent?
    c. Are there enough data to be significant?
    d. Are relevant problem-solving tools being used properly?
    e. Is team interpreting data correctly?
2. Review workplan
    a. Are team members completing tasks effectively and on schedule?
    b. Is there evidence of potential to achieve goal?
    c. Has work plan been modified to reflect any necessary changes to achieve goal?
3. Assess team dynamics
    a. Are team members willing and able to take actions?
    b. Are personnel issues being raised and addressed?
    c. Is team getting the necessary cooperation and support, or is it working on this?

With Sponsor
1. Review the goal and work plan and provide necessary support
2. Send out a memo asking the team to present to the management

improvement, (3) apply the PDCA model, and (4) understand the problem-solving methodology.

Step 1: Do Preliminary Work

Preparatory materials are required for this step.

1. Kickoff meeting.
    a. Facilitator task list for breakthrough kickoff preparation.
    b. Suggested agenda for breakthrough team sessions.
    c. Example memos for invitation to breakthrough team.

T A B L E   12–2

Checklist for Documenting New Procedures and Communicating Progress

With Team Leader and Team
1. Review progress
   a. Are all work plan actions completed by due dates?
   b. Do data show definite progress toward achieving goal?
   c. Are any new activities necessary to achieve goal?
   d. Are all remaining obstacles (physical and psychological) discussed and actions to overcome them set in motion?
   e. Does team sense that efforts are paying off?
2. Document changes, including process and procedure changes documented by team leader
3. Communicate progress to sponsor and senior management, including:
   a. Progress against the goal
   b. Potential economic impact
   c. Changes in process and procedures already implemented
   d. Remaining obstacles

With Sponsor and Senior Management
1. Discuss potential rewards
2. Solicit feedback from team
3. Discuss plans for wrap-up and expansion

2. Team follow-ups.
   a. Checklists for at least a two-week follow-up (allow for feedback).
   b. Checklist for at least a six-week follow-up (allow for feedback and make sure that corrective action items have been addressed from previous review).
   c. Provide appropriate information to the lead quality assurance (LQA) for presentation.
3. Team wrap-up.
   a. Checklist for team wrap-up (how to bring the project to closure and move to another one).
   b. Standardize the project summary form.
   c. Standardize the expansion plan form if applicable.

T A B L E   12–3

Checklist for Achieving Goal and Planning Expansion

With Team Leader and Team

1. Celebrate success
2. Document improvement (a summary report is necessary)
3. Collect and bind all information (work plans, check sheets, process flow charts, fishbone diagrams, etc.)
4. Present results to all interested parties. Presentation should include the following:
   a. Statement of goal
   b. Team members' names and positions
   c. Results
   d. Key actions, including a priority analysis and the economic impact of the actions, key barriers to actions, an assessment of what worked well and what could have been done better, and new processes and procedures implemented
   e. Overall learning
   f. Plans for institutionalization and expansion
5. Plan for future actions (a future plan report is necessary)

With Sponsor and Management

1. Give feedback and rewards to successful teams
2. Discuss expansion and next opportunities

Before kickoff of the project, the facilitator's tasks are as follows:

1. Discuss and understand opportunity area or areas.
2. Agree on the date and agenda for the team kickoff.
3. Assist management in preparation of the invitation to teams.
4. Schedule the orientation session for the team.
5. Schedule the introduction of the opportunity to the team by management.
6. Follow-up with team leader and team members.
7. Prepare equipment and materials for orientation session (overhead projector, at least two flip charts, at least three different color markers in working condition, and VCR and television in working condition if needed).

Preparation of a kickoff meeting agenda also is part of the necessary preliminary work. This meeting must be scheduled sequentially, and the timing must be tailored to fit team schedules over a maximum of three days. This timing is important to sustain the enthusiasm and commitment of both management and team members. Therefore, a kickoff meeting may be scheduled in three sessions. Typically, the first session lasts three hours and covers the team orientation process, with an overview of the team strategy and the opportunity to be resolved. It also includes a visit to the area where the opportunity exists. The second session, usually lasting three and one-half hours, covers the team work group, including crystallization of the goal and the work plan for achieving it. The final session, which may last two hours, covers the clean-up process (tying up loose ends and meeting with the sponsor and team leader to discuss agreement of the goal or goals) and prepares the team for the presentation by the LQA. A typical agenda for this meeting is shown in Table 12–4.

Step 2: Introduce Concept of Continuous Improvement

A management executive usually opens the session. The focus is to introduce the concept of continuous improvement and to communicate the commitment of all the management team for this program. The presentation of the executive is usually no longer than 5 to 10 minutes and covers at least the following thoughts:

> "Over the past few months, you probably have heard a lot about continuous improvement. The TQM approach is a way for teams like yours to move quickly into action on an important improvement opportunity to help your department become a continuously improving organization.
>
> "TQM teams have been launched in many healthcare facilities around the country with some spectacular results (*be specific*). We anticipate the same positive results in our facilities.
>
> "I want to assure you that once the program is under way, we will provide you with additional training and resources as needed. Also, as TQM is being implemented throughout our organization, you will hear others talk about their successes and failures. Please do not discourage these discussions, as they offer an op-

T A B L E   12–4

Agenda for Kickoff Meeting Sessions

Action	End Products	Timing
Session 1: Team Orientation		
Orientation	Team members understand why they were selected	2 hours
■ Management introduction and strategy overview	■ Team members understand strategy	
■ Implementation at work stations; start process flow diagram and cause-and-effect diagram	■ High-level process flow diagram and cause-and-effect diagram	
Visit department with the opportunity	Understand the department work process	30–60 minutes
Total time		**2½–3 hours**
Session 2: Team Work Group and Plan		
Complete high-level process flow	High-level process flow diagram	20 minutes
Complete cause-and-effect diagram	Cause-and-effect diagram	20 minutes
Set goal(s)	Statement of goal(s)	45 minutes
Refine process flow and cause-and-effect diagrams	Complete process flow and cause-and-effect diagrams	30 minutes
Create work plan	Detailed work plan	90 minutes
■ Review cause-and-effect diagram		
■ Brainstorm ideas		
■ In the process use 7 tools		
Total time		**3 hours 25 minutes**
Session 3: Clean-Up Process and Preparation for LQA Presentation		
Help team leader complete work plan and structure analyses	Completed work plan, clear direction for analyses, clear next steps	60 minutes
Schedule follow-up meeting	Date and time for first follow-up	15 minutes
Facilitator and team leader meet with management to review goal and plan	Management is fully briefed on team goal and work plan	60 minutes
Total time		**2 hours 15 minutes**

portunity to learn. At this point, I want to turn over the meeting to your facilitator (*name*), who will formally introduce the TQM strategy."

The facilitator then takes over and gives an overview of the concept. Some of the key items covered in the facilitator's presentation follow these guidelines:

"A continuously improving organization is one that captures opportunities on an ongoing basis while building skills and confidence and instilling a readiness to embrace change to the employees. We hope that our facility has done some of this already, but we all know that every department is acting as though it were the only one that has implemented these techniques. We hope that this TQM strategy not only will provide a consistency between departments but also will achieve short-term performance gains and long-term continuous improvement.

"In this presentation we will introduce this strategy and provide some examples of its use. Let me reiterate that our overall objective is to build a continuously improving organization with small-scale successes over time (of course, the major changes are OK, too). Periodically, a larger scale success will improve performance significantly in a short time frame.

"To be effective in this endeavor, everyone in our organization must be involved. The best way to do this is through teams. Teams are the fundamental vehicle for continuous improvement. Generally speaking, departmental teams achieve many small-scale successes over longer periods of time and are the basic building blocks of continuous improvement. Cross-functional teams convene periodically and tend to create significant impact when the opportunity avails itself but are ad hoc in nature."

The TQM strategy is centered around achieving and building on small-scale, immediate-performance successes, which are keys to the success of the business (called breakthroughs). The vehicle used to pursue these opportunities is teams assembled and empowered to set and tackle short-term goals. There are at least three aims of this strategy:

1. The first is to break through "normal" levels of performance and achieve new levels of performance. Each change focuses on achieving a very specific, razor-sharp goal. The attainment of the goal is very important. It is the accomplishment of this goal that people most frequently talk about, with a good deal of pride on the part of participants.

2. The strategy is not only about achieving the goal. Next, teams must build the skills, procedures, and working methods to sustain progress. No organization is interested in short-term performance hits. Rather, teams must make changes that will sustain progress over the long haul. By the conclusion of each project, each team has made sure that the organization has the capacity to continue making headway.

3. Next, and perhaps most importantly, breakthroughs also help build the readiness and capacity to manage change. By actually achieving an important goal, teams learn a good deal about what's needed to bring about meaningful change. And with success behind them, people are much more ready to participate in change efforts.

Breakthrough Strategy Characteristics

The breakthrough strategy may be summarized in the following:

breakthrough strategy

Achieving and building on small-scale, immediate-performance successes by empowering teams to pursue opportunities that are tied to key business issues.

The results are new performance levels; new skills, procedures, and working methods; and increased readiness and capacity to manage change (the capacity, confidence, and momentum to achieve more).

So, what are the characteristics of breakthrough strategy? There are a number of characteristics that distinguish themselves from other performance improvement programs. First, the strategy itself is goal oriented. Achievements are measured quantifiably against goals developed early in the process. A plan of actions, *not recommendations*, is developed and implemented over a period of six to eight weeks. This quick time frame allows participants to experience success and build momentum toward larger organizational objectives. Finally, the breakthrough strategy is focused on bottom-line performance results. Rather than investing significant amounts of time and resources up front for training and establishing a program, breakthrough focuses on performance and strives for results that will improve that performance.

Step 3: Apply PDCA Model to the Application

The breakthrough strategy is an adaptation of the PDCA model developed by Deming more than 30 years ago. Its concept is as follows:

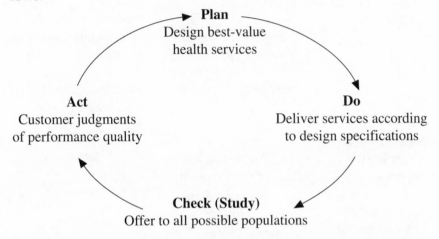

Plan
Design best-value
health services

Act
Customer judgments
of performance quality

Do
Deliver services according
to design specifications

Check (Study)
Offer to all possible populations

Dr. Deming's model broadly outlines the process for continually improving organizations. The "Plan" step identifies opportunities for performance improvement in an organization. Most importantly, the PDCA cycle addresses the idea of experimental change in the "Do" step and then evaluation of those changes during the "Check" step. Using this technique, organizations can try out changes before actually implementing them into day-to-day operations. The "Act" step is the institutionalization of changes.

In real-world application, the breakthrough process maps the PDCA model into six steps, which when followed by organizations have proved to be extremely powerful. The steps are: *Plan*—Identify the opportunity, assemble and empower the team, and define a sharply focused goal; *Do*—problem solve and create a work plan; *Check (Study)*—move into action; and *Act*—institutionalize and expand.

A typical generic application of time model is the following:

Plan

Define opportunity	Define and empower the team	Define *the* goal

Key steps:

Management sponsor or team identifies initial opportunity	Sponsor selects team leader and agrees on opportunity. Team leader collects preparatory data to sharpen opportunity. Sponsor presents opportunity to team.	Conduct preliminary problem solving. Review preparatory analysis. Develop process flow diagram. Develop cause-and-effect diagram. Set breakthrough goal.

Supporting steps:

Team leader reviews opportunity with lead quality assurance and LQA appoints facilitator if needed.
LQA defines opportunity if needed.

Facilitator and team leader plan launch:

- Identify team members.
- Schedule orientation.
- Develop announcement memo (Table 12–5).

Conduct review presentations (Table 12–6).

Do

Problem solve and create work plan

Key steps:

- Conduct detailed problem solving.
- Refine process flow and cause-and-effect diagrams.

T A B L E   12–5

Sample Invitation to Become a Team Member

To: Name of Employee

From: Team sponsor

Subject: Invitation to participate in a total quality management (TQM) team

Date:

I am sure by now you have heard how other organizations, including those in healthcare, have improved the quality of their products and services and improved their performance as well.

Although we are the market leader in our business, competition is stiff. We cannot sit still. We must find ways to help our staff at all levels to find new and better ways of doing things. At its most recent meeting, the executive board, with the approval of the board of trustees, made a commitment to launch a continuous improvement process across our facility. The purpose of this process is to structure an environment in which all of us can contribute to continually improving our performance.

I would like to invite you to help us get started by participating on a departmental TQM team. As a team member, you will be asked to help identify and realize improvements in your department within 6–8 weeks.

You will be given plenty of assistance along the way, including training in some key analytic tools to help you diagnose issues in your department and find solutions. The corporate quality facilitator (*name*) from our training department will help in this process and will be actively involved. Whenever necessary, outside consultants will be used for specific tasks.

The project will kick off on (*date*) at (*time*) in (*location*). This first meeting will take about (*X*) hours. In preparation for this project, please consider these questions:

What products or services does your department produce?

Who are your customers, both internal and/or external?

What specifically is most important to your customers?

What do you believe are the most significant areas for improving performance provided to your customers?

I look forward to seeing you on (*date*). Please let me know if you have any questions before then.

Sincerely,

(*signature and title*)

T A B L E   12–6

Sample Memo for TQM Project Review

To: TQM team leaders
From: Team sponsor
Subject: TQM project review
Date:

Our TQM teams are a very important experiment for us in learning how to build an organization focused on continuous performance improvement. To update the management team on your progress, I would like to invite you and your team (if possible) to make a 15- to 20-minute presentation to the Lead Quality Assurance on your project.

Please include the following in your presentation:

1. Your goal and why you chose it.
2. List of team members.
3. Your work plan and what you accomplished so far.
4. Any results to date toward your goal.
5. Results of analysis you conducted (e.g., cause-and-effect diagram, process flow chart, Pareto chart).
6. Obstacles you encountered or expect to encounter.
7. Any anticipated help needed.

I look forward to hearing your progress.

Sincerely,
(*signature and title*)

- Structure analysis and data collection.
- Create work plan.

Supporting steps:
Commit to goal. Team leader reviews goal and plan with sponsor and revises if needed.

Check (Study)
Move into action

Key steps:

- Implement work plan.
- Meet and revise work plan as needed.

Supporting steps:

- Conduct review or progress with facilitator at specified intervals.
- Review with LQA.
- Conduct review with sponsor at specified intervals or as needed.

Act
Institutionalize and expand

Key steps:

- Institutionalize change.
- Agree on measures to monitor on ongoing basis.
- Develop expansion plan and plan next project.

Supporting steps:
Conduct review with facilitator at predetermined intervals.

Step 4: Understand the Problem-Solving Methodology

Before we attack the problem, we must understand it and formalize the actions to be taken. A typical breakthrough process can be divided into six steps: (1) identify an improvement opportunity, (2) assemble and empower a team, (3) set the goals, (4) collect and analyze data, (5) achieve the goal, and (6) diffuse the results to other areas.

Identify an Improvement Opportunity
A senior executive often begins the breakthrough process by identifying an urgent and compelling improvement opportunity. To get the process under way, there must be a set of criteria. The criteria generally follow the following guidelines.

Urgent and Compelling Opportunity   People almost always have more than enough work to do and opportunities to tackle. Therefore, we want to work only on the things that count and will make a real difference. Teams work on those issues that are most central to the organization's success and are a priority for the organization.

Performance Driven   Not preparatory activities or programs. Since we are trying to achieve performance successes, teams focus directly on specific, measurable results. As a result, within a short time, the team will be able to demonstrate with hard data whether it achieved a success. While installing programs and other preparatory activities can be good things to do, they do not necessarily give people the same positive reinforcement, which is so central to the breakthrough strategy.

Significant Progress Achievable in a Short Time
The breakthrough strategy aims to help energize change efforts. It has been found that people respond most positively to more immediate performance challenges. Therefore, a key criterion is to work on projects for which significant progress can be made within six to eight weeks, rather than a number of months or longer.

Affected Staff Willing to Change   Rather than starting with opportunities to which there may be a good deal of resistance, we are looking for opportunities, locations, and people with readiness for change. Why start where there is resistance, when there are so many opportunities to tap into people's readiness for improvement?

Results Achievable with Existing Resources and Authority   To achieve results within a short time, it is important that the team not need additional resources and authority that could take quite a while to receive. Also, it is too easy in change efforts to point to all the things that others need to do before improvement can happen. Therefore, strong emphasis is placed on teams making progress with the resources and authority they already have that may not be fully tapped. Do not expect to have others change to make the goal. First, do the best you can, with what you have, and then look at others. The clue to success is specificity. The more specific you are, the more likely the team will be successful.

Assemble and Empower a Team
The composition and expectation of the team is crucial to the success of the project. Therefore, these questions must be asked:

Are the right people involved? Are there key skills or pieces of information the team will need that someone has? Will pursuing the opportunity change someone's work process substantially? Is there someone who is a possible roadblock or champion? Will the team function well together? Are there personality differences to overcome?

Does the team have the authority and ability to address the opportunity? Again, are the right people on the team? Is the team ready to address the opportunity?

Does the team have support from management?

Is the team willing to work to overcome resistance? Is it prepared for some resistance?

Does the entire team buy into (have ownership in) the goal?

Barriers to Change   One can see that these questions—although simple and straightforward—may represent a change in the status quo. Change is threatening, and consequently people protect themselves with either psychological or organizational barriers to change or a combination of both. If you were to ask people to identify what needs to be done for the organization to achieve higher levels of performance, how many times do people say things similar to the following? "If only I were a more effective leader or manager . . ." "If only I could get people motivated . . ." "If only I were better organized . . ." "If only I could run more effective meetings . . ." The answer is rarely, if ever, "I can help." Instead, we tend to look outside ourselves to identify what needs to change to improve performance. This is a human response. Why? Because we protect ourselves from anxiety created by demands for change. These mechanisms are sophisticated and diverse. We all have them. The key is to identify how these may be operating within ourselves and the people with whom we work. What makes this particularly difficult is that in some cases each of these barriers can be true. People are doing all they can, someone else may have to change, and more resources may be needed. (Appendix C provides a list of some of the barriers that one may encounter during the implementation process.) The trick is to identify when these represent actual rather than psychological barriers.

Some examples of psychological barriers are as follows:

Psychological Barriers
- The patients won't like that.
- We are not allowed to do that.
- Our facilities are unique. We do not do it any other way.
- Give me more people, time, budget, and so on.
- We always have done it that way.
- The physicians won't do that.
- I am doing all I can.
- All I do is straighten out the other guy.
- That is not really a problem.
- We have tried things like that before. It won't work here.

There are also organizational barriers that limit performance. These barriers are real and keep performance at so-called normal levels. We need to overcome these barriers by using a structured process, which focuses on a razor-sharp, measurable goal; a written work plan specifying people's responsibilities; and regular progress reviews. Some examples of organizational barriers are:

Organizational Barriers
- Goals are too many, too far out in the future, vague, or unmeasurable.
- Fuzzy accountability. Who will do what by when?
- Daily operating pressures prevent management from inviting people to participate.
- Inadequate information, training, tools, and so on.
- Sacred cows.

The breakthrough strategy helps overcome both types of barriers. First, senior management's support creates urgency and makes it easier to cut the red tape. Second, team members know quickly whether or not they have accomplished their goal. Finally, working as a team helps individuals develop the confidence to overcome barriers.

Set the Goal
Setting the goal, including the level of accomplishment to be achieved, reinforces the commitment to goal achievement. The goals set by the team must meet at least the following criteria.

A Step Up in Performance   The objective of the break-through goal is to challenge the team to perform at a level higher than it has in the past.

Measurable, Quantifiable, Bottom-Line Results Oriented   Because we are trying to achieve performance successes, teams focus directly on specific, measurable results, so that within a short time they will know whether they have achieved a success. As mentioned earlier, although installing training and awareness programs and other preparatory activities can be good things to do, they do not necessarily give people the same positive reinforcement upon accomplishment, which is central to the break-through strategy. Generally, these types of activities do not actually produce a performance result.

Necessary Resources and Authority under the Control or Influence of Team   To achieve results within a short time, it is important that the team not need additional resources and authority that could take quite a while to receive. Also, it is too easy in change efforts to point to all the things that others need to do before improvement can happen. Therefore, strong emphasis is placed on teams making progress with the resources and authority they already have that may not be fully tapped.

Identify the Opportunity with Greatest Potential for Impact   The team should have a sense for the scale of the potential impact associated with the piece of the opportunity they elect to address. Those with the greatest potential impact should be addressed first.

Achievable in a Short Time   The breakthrough strategy aims to help energize efforts at change. It has been found that people respond most positively to more immediate performance challenges. Therefore, a key criterion is to work on projects where significant progress can be made within six to eight weeks, rather than a number of months or longer. This point is of paramount importance since it implies that, unless excellent communication channels exist in the organization, the time limitations may prove unreachable. This is the Demand Triangle, which is shown in

Figure 12–1. The characteristic of this triangle is that the manager, sponsor, and team leader have opened the links of communication toward the facilitator. In fact, their facilitator is aware of their availability to help.

Agreed On or Committed to by Team   This process is based on mutual accountability. The team can be held accountable only if they have agreed on the goal.

Collect and Analyze Data

To accomplish the goal, the team uses both qualitative and quantitative problem-solving tools to diagnose the problem and generate solutions (Figures 12–2, 12–3, and 12–4). The team then develops a detailed work plan to follow. The idea here is not so much to accomplish the goal by working together, but rather to find innovative ways to work smarter. Because this is the heart of the breakthrough strategy, we are presenting the problem-solving approach in a detailed outline format.

FIGURE   12–1

Demand Triangle

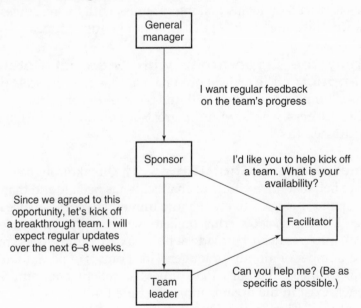

FIGURE   12-2

Sample Brainstorming Form to Create a Work Plan

Action Items		
Analyses to Do, Baseline Data to Collect Tools to Use	Changes in Policies, Procedures, Scheduling, Work Flow	Communications with and Involvement of Shifts, Departments, Managers to Share Information and Build

F I G U R E   12–3

Goal Achievement Status Form

Department: _____   Date: _____

Goal just achieved:

Data to collect and review so that we maintain our improvement:

Data to collect	Frequency of collection/review	Person responsible for review

---

Expansion opportunities (how we can do even better on this goal, or how we can expand it in our own department or to other departments):

Possible new breakthrough opportunities in this department:

Actions to take or data to collect before next meeting:

Action	Person responsible	End date

Next team meeting date:

F I G U R E   12–4

Project Summary Report

Date: _____

Project start date: _____   Project end date: _____

Department: _____

Opportunity area: _____

Goal:

Result:

Team leader:
Team members:

Team actions (three to five major actions taken by the team—from the work plan):

Pending actions of the team, if any:

Team accomplishments:
Service benefits to customer (internal and external):

Improved teamwork/communication/morale:

Financial benefits:

I. *Prerequisites to problem solving*
  A. What is a problem?
    1. A problem is a symptom, not a cause or a solution.
    2. A problem is a gap between what is happening and what you want to happen.
    3. A problem is something that keeps you from achieving your goal.
    4. A problem could be a defect, an error, a missed deadline, a lost opportunity, or an inefficient operation.
    5. A problem may be thought of as an opportunity.
  B. What is the road to continuous improvement?
    1. TQM and problem solving: Problem solving is an important activity for attaining continuous process improvement.
    2. Kaizen and breakthroughs: Kaizen is a gradual, relentless, incremental process improvement over time, whereas breakthrough is a sudden, significant improvement in process performance achieved in a short time. Continuous process improvement is best achieved by a combination of both Kaizen and breakthroughs. Ideally, an organization should employ and encourage both Kaizen and breakthrough in its improvement strategy.
  C. What are chronic versus sporadic problems?
    1. A sporadic problem is a sudden, elevated departure of the level of a problem from its historic, status quo level.
    2. A chronic problem is the difference between the historic level and an optimum or zero level; a chronic problem is a chronic "disease" that can economically be eliminated.
  D. What are three typical responses to problems?
    1. View them as burdens.
    2. Ignore them.
    3. Accept them as challenges or opportunities to improve.

    E. What are the nine roadblocks to effective problem solving?
1. Lack of time.
2. Lack of ownership in the problem.
3. Lack of recognition of the problem.
4. A belief that errors have become a way of life.
5. Ignorance of the importance of a problem.
6. A belief that no one can do anything about some problems.
7. A poor balance by upper management among cost, schedule, and quality.
8. Fearful people who try to protect themselves and are afraid to rock the boat.
9. Blame by management.

    F. What are the six key ingredients required to correct problems?
1. Awareness of the importance of eliminating errors and the cost of errors to the business.
2. A desire to eliminate errors.
3. Training provided in proven, effective methods for solving and preventing problems.
4. Analysis of failures to identify and correct the real root causes of problems.
5. Follow-up in tracking problems and action commitments.
6. Recognition, which gives liberal credit to all those who participate.

    G. What must management provide?
1. A motivating environment conducive to effective, companywide problem solving.
2. A real opportunity for problem solving.
3. A systematic approach (road map) for effective problem solving.
4. Knowledge of the tools for problem solving.

II. *Problem-solving cycle*

    A. Why use a structured problem-solving approach? A structured, systematic, problem-solving approach:
1. Illustrates the relative *importance* of problems.
2. Shows the real *root causes* of problems.

3. Helps problem solvers get *unstuck*, knows *where* they are at, keeps them on *track*, and *perseveres* to get results.
4. Helps keep problems solved.
5. Establishes *accountability* and a *motivating* environment for problem solving.
6. Produces consistently *better* solutions to problems than do unstructured approaches.

B. A typical five-step problem-solving (opportunity) cycle:
  1. Select the problem that represents an error, waste, bottleneck in a specific area, and so on. The process of selection is as follows:
     a) Prepare a problem list.
     b) Collect data to determine the magnitude of each problem.
     c) Prioritize the problems to determine which problems should be worked on first. Almost always, a vital few problems account for the greatest proportion of the losses.
     d) Select the target problem, generally the problem whose solution will have the greatest beneficial impact.
     e) Prepare a specific problem statement (e.g., reduce medication errors from 19 percent to 5 percent in the next six months). The statement will represent the specific problem assignment or project committed to.
  2. Find the root cause. This analysis step is usually the crucial work of the project. Problems must be solved at the level of the root cause if they are to remain fully and permanently corrected. The actual process is as follows:
     a) Identify all the possible causes of the problem using brainstorming, cause-and-effect diagrams, and so on.
     b) If necessary, collect data to ascertain the failure mechanism using check sheets, frequency diagrams, and so on.

   c) Select the most likely cause using a Pareto
      analysis or other quality tool.
3. Correct the problem. The idea here is to follow a
   plan that will eliminate the problem or at least
   reduce it to a level compatible with the team's
   goal. The process for doing so is the following:
   a) Make a temporary fix, if appropriate, to
      protect the customer until a permanent fix can
      be implemented.
   b) Develop alternative solutions for correcting
      the problem.
   c) Select the best possible solution by narrowing
      down the alternatives using a priority-setting
      approach and making a final, consensus
      decision.
   d) Develop an implementation action plan,
      which includes a time schedule for
      implementation. Everyone who is involved in
      carrying out the solution should be consulted
      and should approve the plan. The plan should
      answer these basic questions: Who? What?
      Where? When? How?
   e) Establish the method for measuring the
      success of the proposed solution. Remember,
      the criterion for success was established as
      part of the problem statement in step 1.
   f) Gain management approval, if necessary, for
      implementation.
   g) Implement the action plan.
4. Verify correction. This is a step that uses the
   criteria for success established in step 1 and the
   measuring method established in step 3 to verify
   the goal or goals. The actual process of verification
   is as follows:
   a) Measure the impact of the solution.
   b) Make a decision. Is the problem solved to a
      level compatible with the team's goal? Have
      any unforeseen new problems been created by
      the solution?

    c) If the correction is unsatisfactory, the team must go back to an earlier step, selecting an alternative solution or possibly even selecting an alternative root cause, then proceeding.

    d) If the correction is satisfactory, any temporary protective fix should be removed.

5. Prevent recurrence . . . then recycle. This is an often overlooked aspect of problem solving, the benefits of which cannot be overstated. The actual process is as follows:

    a) Develop innovative methods for proofing the system for mistakes.

    b) Alter systems and procedures to reflect the new, optimal practices.

    c) Train all involved personnel in the new methods.

    d) Publicize the results. Apply the knowledge gained to the rest of the organization with similar conditions.

    e) Continue to monitor the problem.

    f) Recognize the team's success.

    g) Prepare a final project report and/or management presentation, which describes the problem, methods used to correct it, and quality productivity gains achieved.

    h) Recycle. Once the five steps of the problem-solving cycle have been completed, the team should return to step 1, select another significant problem for correction, and continue improvement efforts. This simple problem-solving process is both easy to understand and to remember. However, to be effective, each of the steps must be fully completed before the next step is begun. The reader is warned to pay attention to the fact that there are several iteration or feedback loops that may have to be followed to properly complete the cycle. A step should not be considered complete until the final substep is carried out.

C. Tools of quality:
   1. Teams need to learn and apply a number of
      quality tools (analytic techniques) to aid them in
      their working through the five steps of the
      problem-solving cycle. These tools are primarily
      used for collecting, analyzing, and understanding
      data or other information.
   2. Quality tools inventory:
      a) Numerous quality tools may be applied to
         problem solving. Some of these are complex,
         advanced, mathematical techniques, whereas
         others are simple to learn and apply. Each of
         the tools has advantages and disadvantages,
         and proper training is therefore required for
         their use.
      b) Of the plethora of quality tools, seven tools are
         widely considered to be the basic tools of
         quality. They are:
         (1) Flowchart
         (2) Check sheet
         (3) Histogram
         (4) Pareto chart
         (5) Cause-and-effect (fishbone) diagram
         (6) Scatter diagram
         (7) Control chart
         These tools are easy to learn by everyone in
         the organization. They are effective in
         achieving success in basic problem solving
         and are essential to any properly designed
         improvement strategy (see Chapter 6).
      c) The team's appropriate use of the seven basic
         tools in the healthcare environment will
         require considerable practice and experience.
         Patience and perseverance become important
         virtues; they will pay off!
D. Process improvement cycle:
   1. Why a structured process improvement approach?
      A structured, systematic, process improvement
      approach:
      a) Provides a more tightly focused process than

the problem-solving cycle, concentrating on improving the quality of a single process output (product or service).

b) Lends itself especially well to customer issues, since it builds and strengthens ties between customer and supplier.

c) Provides a catalyst for never-ending improvement through its continuous refocusing on customer needs and expectations.

d) Affords a prime opportunity to use statistical process control (SPC) methods for process analysis, control, and improvement.

e) Focuses improvement efforts on both product/service quality and waste reduction.

f) Provides to improvement teams an enhanced motivational environment for their improvement efforts.

2. 14-step process improvement cycle:

a) Step 1. Identify the output.

(1) Prepare a statement that answers the question, What is to be done? It should consist of two parts: a tangible, specific noun followed by a verb describing what you do to produce the output.

(2) The statement should be neither too broad nor too specific if it is to be useful.

(3) Examples: medication delivered; patient prepared for surgery; order shipped; report typed.

b) Step 2. Identify the customer.

(1) The primary customer is the next person in the work process, the person who will receive your output as input and will act on it.

(2) The customer may be either external or internal.

(3) Secondary customers and end users may be identified if their requirements are of significance.

c) Step 3. Identify the customer requirements.
   (1) What does the customer want, need, or
       expect of the output?
   (2) Customer requirements may be general or
       specific.
   (3) Customer requirements often fall into
       categories such as cost, accuracy,
       timeliness, quantity, completeness,
       dimension, performance, and appearance.
   (4) Supplier–customer interaction is essential.
       Both customer and supplier specify,
       negotiate, and evaluate information before
       reaching an agreement.
   (5) Examples: Report needed ASAP; expense
       cannot exceed the budget; colors must
       match; quick response time needed.
d) Step 4. Translate requirements into product or
   service specifications.
   (1) Customer's needs are put into language
       that reflects the supplier's active
       participation.
   (2) Specifications should be measurable,
       realistic, and achievable and should be
       reviewed with the customer to be certain
       both parties understand and agree what
       the output should be.
   (3) Examples: Eyeglasses needed by 4 P.M.
       Friday; weight 400 pounds maximum;
       typing double-spaced.
e) Step 5. Identify the work process.
   (1) What are the process elements? A
       Fishbone diagram used as a process
       analysis map may help to identify the
       equipment, people, input, methods, and
       environmental factors in the work process.
   (2) List step-by-step what must be done to
       achieve the output. Flowcharts are
       especially helpful here.
   (3) Identify or develop the needed
       documentation, which describes or

provides instructions for the work process.

f) Step 6. Select the process measurables and measurement.

  (1) Select the critical measurements for the process output. These measurements should be derived from customer requirements and product specifications and should permit an objective evaluation of the quality of output.

  (2) Measurements should provide for early identification of potential and actual problems, where stress is on the prevention rather than on the detection of errors or defects.

  (3) Examples: Weight in grams; transit time in minutes; response time in seconds.

  (4) Also, select measurements for key:

    (a) Process inputs, such as raw materials, incoming items, energy, supplies, and information.

    (b) In-process factors (intermediate process outputs): in-process conditions that have an impact on the process output, such as temperature, pressure, and time.

    (c) Process performance criteria, such as scrap, rework, downtime, yield, delays, and efficiency.

  (5) These measurements become the basis for process analysis, control, and improvement.

g) Step 7. Determine the process capability.

  (1) This step helps determine if the existing process can produce an output that consistently meets the agreed-to product specifications with minimal waste.

  (2) The process is operated according to standard practices; output measurement

data are collected and analyzed to provide a statistical evaluation of process control (consistency) and process capability (ability to meet specifications).

(3) This step is an important activity of SPC.

h) Step 8. Decide if the process is capable.

(1) If the evaluation indicates that specifications are *not* being met consistently and that excessive waste (scrap, rework, delays, errors, etc.) is experienced, the work process must be revamped or improved. This requires problem solving; proceed to step 9.

(2) If the process capability assessment of step 7 determines that the existing process *can* produce an output that consistently meets specification requirements and does so with minimal waste, proceed to step 10 to produce the output.

i) Step 9. Problem solve to improve the work process.

(1) Use the five-step problem-solving cycle to revamp or improve the existing process.

(2) If the process capability problem indicated in step 7 is a lack of process control (instability or inconsistency), indicated by sporadic deviations of the process average from the target, status quo, or historic level, the solution is one of identifying the destabilizing (special/assignable) causes and eliminating them. After special-cause problem solving is completed, loop back to steps 7 and 8 (reassess process control). If the problem is solved, proceed to step 10; if not, continue to repeat the cycle at step 9 as needed, until process control is achieved.

(3) If the process capability problem indicated in step 7 is an *inherent* inability to meet

specification requirements, the process system must be fundamentally changed. This requires identifying those key process factors (common or random causes) which have a major impact on the quality of process output and modifying them and their effects. After common-cause problem solving is completed, loop back to step 5 to redefine the revised work process and proceed. If at steps 7 and 8 the process capability problem is solved, proceed to step 10; if not, continue to repeat the cycle at step 9 as needed, until process capability is achieved.

(4) If repeated attempts still leave you with an incapable process, talk with the customer who needs to know what to expect. A renegotiation of the requirements may be possible. If not, the customer may want to find another supplier.

j) Step 10. Produce the output, continuing to follow the standard practices (or the newly established practices, which should be standardized for the new, revamped process).

k) Step 11. Evaluate the results.

(1) Evaluation of results must be based on the product specifications that both customer and supplier agreed to as part of step 4. Those specifications are a template against which results are compared.

(2) There is a major difference between this step and step 7 (determine process capability). Here you are evaluating how well you *actually did* (not how well you are *capable* of doing). The emphasis is on results rather than on process.

(3) There are two potential types of problems at this point:

        (*a*) The product output does not meet specification requirements.

        (*b*) The product output meets specification requirements, but the customer is dissatisfied with the product.

l) Step 12. Decide if there is a problem.

    (1) If the evaluation of step 11 indicates that there is a problem of either type, problem solving must be carried out. Proceed to step 13.

    (2) If no problem exists, continue production and proceed to step 14.

m) Step 13. Problem solve to improve results.

    (1) Use the five-step problem-solving cycle to troubleshoot the problem.

    (2) If the problem with the process output is of type (*a*) (the process output does not meet specification requirements), the cause of the problem is one of nonconformance to standard practices (since the process was shown to be capable in step 7). The solution to this type of problem lies in identifying the nonconforming practice or practices and restoring operations according to established standard practices at step 10.

    (3) If the problem with the process output is of type (*b*) (the product output meets specification requirements, but the customer is dissatisfied with the product), the cause of the problem is usually one of three things:

        (*a*) Improper understanding of customer requirements.

        (*b*) Improper translation of requirements info specifications.

        (*c*) Improper process monitoring (measurement).

Any of these causes requires looping
back to steps 3, 4, or 6 for corrective
action.

n) Step 14. Recycle.

   (1) At this point, there should be no evident
   problems of process capability or results.

   (2) However, there may be opportunities for
   further quality improvement of the
   process output, for example, in terms of
   reduced variability. This could result in
   not merely meeting but in exceeding
   customer expectations.

   (3) Of course, customer needs and
   expectations are rarely static. They are
   likely to change, especially in terms of
   becoming more restrictive.

   (4) These opportunities for continuous
   process improvement require recycling
   back into the process improvement cycle.

   (5) Under any circumstances, continue to
   monitor the work process and the
   results to maintain the required level
   of quality.

3. Problem solving versus process improvement: The
   reader will notice that both the five-step problem
   solving cycle and the 14 steps of the process
   improvement cycle are systematic approaches for
   continuous improvement; more importantly, they
   work in a variety of situations. Both cycles are
   extremely well suited for team-oriented activity.
   However, the dilemma is not whether they are
   friendly toward the user or whether they will
   deliver results. The dilemma is how do we know
   which systematic method to select for appropriate
   use. It is not always obvious which of the two
   methods to use to tackle a particular issue. It takes
   some skill and experience to make the selection.
   Fortunately, no matter which method you select,
   once you start using it you are likely to learn

quickly whether it is helping you to accomplish your objective. The following two items may help in the selection.

a) In general, use the process improvement cycle when you need to improve the quality of a particular, currently existing output or you are about to produce a new output.

b) Use the problem-solving cycle when there is a gap between what is currently happening and what you want to happen. Note that this cycle is an integral part of the process improvement cycle at steps 9 and 13.

A final note about work plans. They are defined actions that the team plans to use in reaching its goal. In some cases, they are individually defined responsibilities that ensure accountability and participation. The specificity may be stated in the form of start and end dates, intermediate checkpoints, and so on. The idea of a work plan is to keep team members informed of progress so necessary actions can be taken. A typical work plan will include:

a) Goal. All involved must be aware of the goal that the team is pursuing.

b) Team leader. The team leader has prime responsibility for the project.

c) Action. What is it that will actually be done? A detailed description of the activity being performed.

d) Responsibility. Establishes who will be responsible for a particular action.

e) Status. Tracks progress that team has made with respect to completed actions.

Achieve the Goal

To achieve breakthrough goals, teams are not asked to work harder or longer. Rather, teams are encouraged to work smarter, to try out innovative approaches that help them perform more effectively. Typical innovations in healthcare are:

Clarify Customer Needs   What does your customer really want? Better quality? Easier access to your service? For example, what time do doctors need to receive the x-ray results? 8 A.M.? Noon? 3 P.M.?

Develop Performance Measurements   We tend to manage what we measure, and often we need to develop new ways to measure performance based on new customer needs. For example, what is our turnaround time in the operating rooms? What is our specimen processing finish time each night?

Empower the Front Line   The principle here is to involve people closest to the front lines in improving performance. For example, employees in the lab should be responsible for identifying innovative approaches for the specimen processing.

Break Down Barriers   Many breakthroughs are successful because groups work together. Once the barriers are broken down, many new ideas may surface. For example, in the process of improving turnaround time for the operating rooms, there must be communication among personnel in scheduling, medical records, x-ray, lab, anesthesiology, and so on.

Eliminate Waste   Waste is everywhere. The issue is not if we have waste but rather how much. It is the responsibility of the team to identify waste and do something about it. For example, in specimen processing, reduce the number of rebags received from customers. Reduce the x-ray reading time. Reduce response time.

Do It Right the First Time   We all say it, but few of us do it. Some of the reasons for not doing it may be lack of time, pressure, resources, and unrealistic expectations. Doing it right the first time may take a little longer but saves enormous amounts of time and money in the long run. For example, read the patient's name tag one more time before surgery; you may prevent a wrong surgery. If you are in doubt about a drug prescription and dosage, verify them with the prescribing doctor; you may prevent a wrong drug reaction or even death.

Process in Parallel   In healthcare we must recognize that the processes often are in parallel. This means that rather than a process working one after another, you try to move downstream activities upstream. In this way groups can work simultaneously rather than wait for another department to complete its work before starting. For example, a patient comes to the emergency department. At that point, the interfacing is a one-to-one relationship between patient and emergency department. However, other departments get into the act very quickly, such as admitting, medical records, x-ray, lab, and respiratory.

Share Service Delivery   This concept means bringing standards and measures to previously unmanaged areas. For example, provide next-day delivery on all routine tests.

Diffuse the Results to Other Areas
Once the breakthrough changes have been made, the team makes permanent changes to the day-to-day operations that institutionalize the improvement they have realized. Those actions that were successful should be introduced to the organization in an ongoing fashion and must be documented. Those that are not successful should be discarded. The team must then turn its attention to what it will do next. Map out a plan for when to meet again and what to take as a breakthrough goal.

There are at least four ways for the team to expand on the initial success. They are:

1. Teams almost always continue to track performance of the initial goal and continue identifying ways to improve on it. Use of the problem-solving tools continues to reveal improvement opportunities to build on initial efforts.
2. Teams also launch efforts aimed at other complementary measures of performance. For example, having reduced error rates, teams can move on to reducing cycle times.
3. To identify additional improvement opportunities, teams can map customer–supplier relationships. This mapping exercise can help reveal potential improvements for new focus or can lead teams to think about reengineering their work process.

4. Another expansion route might be to sponsor cross-functional teams to tackle improvement opportunities that require involvement from other teams. This would be a likely outcome of a customer–supplier mapping exercise. Once the expansion has been determined as a likely program, management may initiate changes in support systems to support continued performance gains. The most likely items are:

   a. Information systems—if teams can identify new kinds of data that would be helpful. For example, a system whereby all medications may be cross-referenced with the patient's medical history.

   b. Training—if new skills are needed to advance performance gain. For example, reengineering training.

   c. Technology—if teams have pushed the limits of existing technology and could benefit from new technological advances. For example, provide personal computers to facilitate the team's efforts.

The issue of implementation and breakthrough in any organization is important. This chapter has focused on just some of the specific items that may benefit TQM implementers. Remember that each organization is unique and presents its own problems. To supplement the discussion, several generic flowcharts are included that give a pictorial view of quality improvement in the organization (Figures 12–5 through 12–13).

F I G U R E   12–5

Quality Improvement (QI) Road Map: Overview

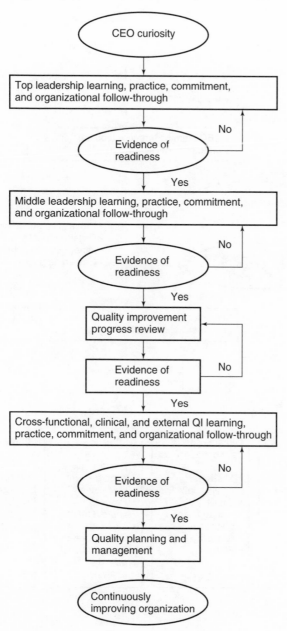

FIGURE 12–6

Quality Improvement (QI) Road Map: Top Leadership

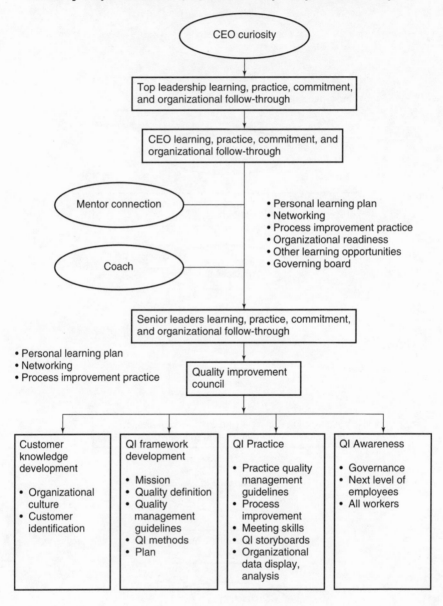

F I G U R E   12–7

Quality Improvement (QI) Road Map:
Top Leadership–Illustrative Evidence

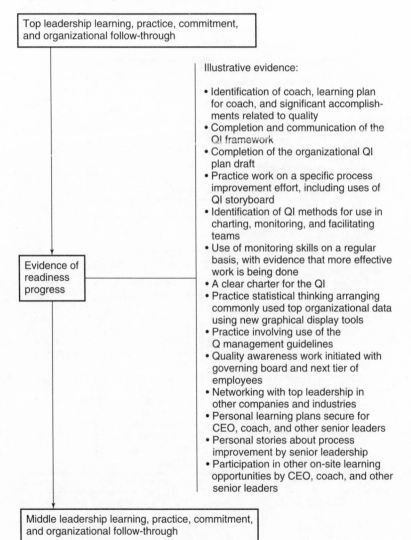

Top leadership learning, practice, commitment, and organizational follow-through

Evidence of readiness progress

Illustrative evidence:

- Identification of coach, learning plan for coach, and significant accomplishments related to quality
- Completion and communication of the QI framework
- Completion of the organizational QI plan draft
- Practice work on a specific process improvement effort, including uses of QI storyboard
- Identification of QI methods for use in charting, monitoring, and facilitating teams
- Use of monitoring skills on a regular basis, with evidence that more effective work is being done
- A clear charter for the QI
- Practice statistical thinking arranging commonly used top organizational data using new graphical display tools
- Practice involving use of the Q management guidelines
- Quality awareness work initiated with governing board and next tier of employees
- Networking with top leadership in other companies and industries
- Personal learning plans secure for CEO, coach, and other senior leaders
- Personal stories about process improvement by senior leadership
- Participation in other on-site learning opportunities by CEO, coach, and other senior leaders

Middle leadership learning, practice, commitment, and organizational follow-through

F I G U R E   12–8

Quality Improvement (QI) Road Map: Middle Leadership

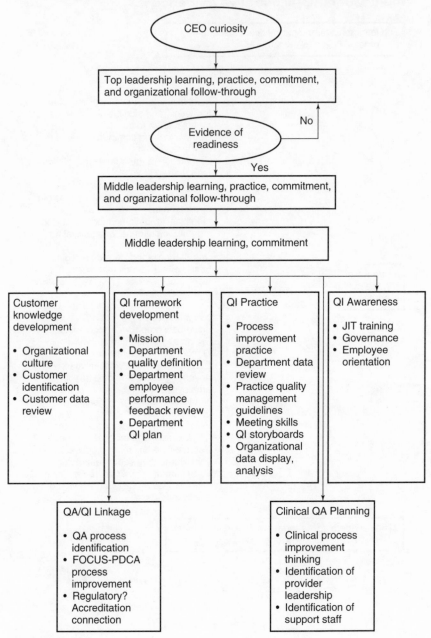

JIT indicates just-in-time.

F I G U R E   12–9

Quality Improvement (QI) Road Map: Middle Leadership–Illustrative Evidence

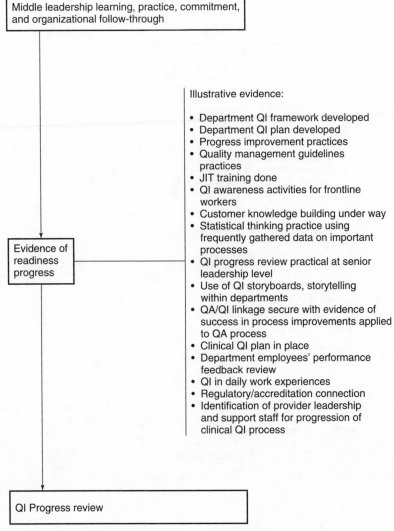

Middle leadership learning, practice, commitment, and organizational follow-through

Illustrative evidence:

- Department QI framework developed
- Department QI plan developed
- Progress improvement practices
- Quality management guidelines practices
- JIT training done
- QI awareness activities for frontline workers
- Customer knowledge building under way
- Statistical thinking practice using frequently gathered data on important processes
- QI progress review practical at senior leadership level
- Use of QI storyboards, storytelling within departments
- QA/QI linkage secure with evidence of success in process improvements applied to QA process
- Clinical QI plan in place
- Department employees' performance feedback review
- QI in daily work experiences
- Regulatory/accreditation connection
- Identification of provider leadership and support staff for progression of clinical QI process

Evidence of readiness progress

QI Progress review

JIT indicates just-in-time; QA, quality assurance.

F I G U R E   12–10

Quality Improvement (QI) Road Map: QI Progress Review

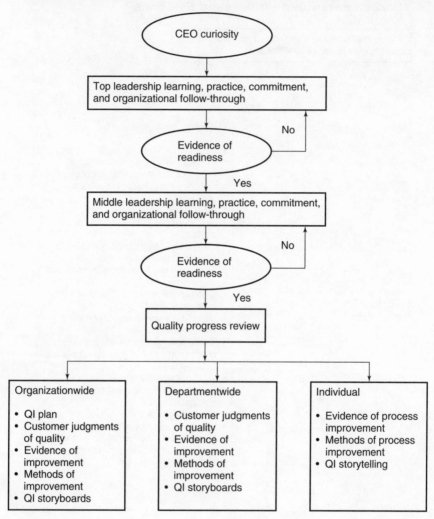

F I G U R E   12-11

Quality Improvement (QI) Road Map:
QI Progress Review—Illustrative Evidence

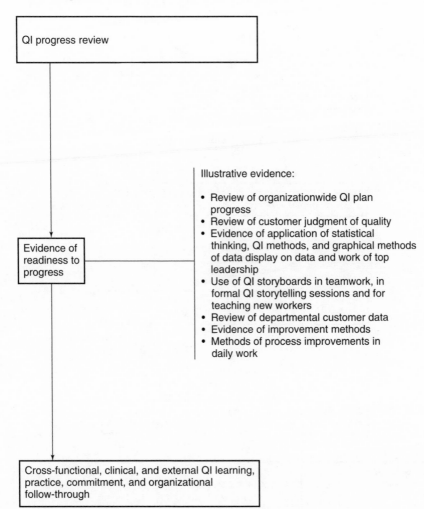

F I G U R E   12–12

Quality Improvement (QI) Road Map: Cross-Functional, Clinical, and External QI

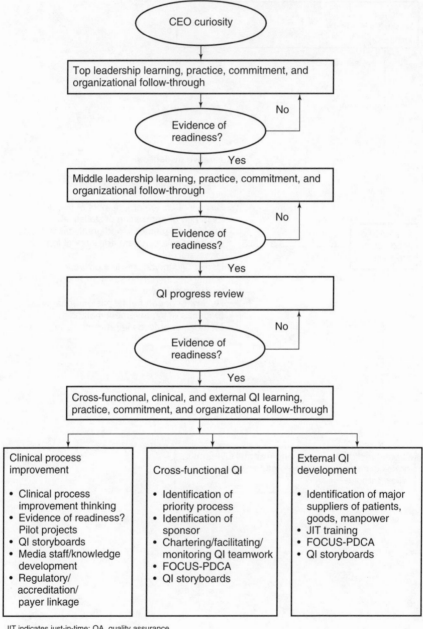

JIT indicates just-in-time; QA, quality assurance.

F I G U R E   1 2 – 1 3

Quality Improvement (QI) Road Map: Cross-Functional, Clinical, and External QI–Illustrative Evidence

Cross-functional, clinical, and external QI learning, practice, commitment, and organizational follow-through

Illustrative evidence:

Clinical

- Evidence of process thinking applied to a clinical process
- Systematic use of one of the suggested methods of clinical process improvement
- Identification of support infrastructures to support physician and other clinician involvement
- Identification and practice by curious physicians of systematic process improvement thinking
- Demonstrated use of QI storyboards to illustrate thought
- Plan for physician education that is related to and built upon the successful elements of the "pilot" educational efforts with early adopters found within the medical staff
- Evidence of link to regulatory and accreditation efforts to minimize duplicative work

Cross-functional

- Evidence of selection process for choosing the first priority process
- Evidence of process to monitor and facilitate the work of teams that cross traditional organizational lines
- Evidence of method to link the external customers of the hospital to the methods of process improvement prioritization
- Methods for JIT training of new team members
- Methods for ensuring that process knowledgeable people are involved
- Evidence that clear planning precedes the formation of team efforts
- Evidence of use of QI storyboards and formalized QI storytelling
- Evidence of use of sponsors

External QI development

- Evidence of method for the identification of major suppliers of patients, human resources, and goods and suppliers
- Evidence of method for the identification and prioritization of processes
- Methods for JIT training
- Method for chartering and monitoring and facilitating jointly conducted QI efforts
- Evidence of use of QI storyboards
- Evidence of improvements made

Evidence of readiness to progress

Quality planning and management

JIT indicates just-in-time; QA, quality assurance.

CHAPTER 13

A Case Study
in Quality Management

REDUCING VIOLENCE IN A HOSPITAL'S
PSYCHIATRIC WARDS

BACKGROUND

XYZ Hospital is a large community hospital, providing medical-surgical, emergency, and mental healthcare. The psychiatric wards accommodate patients for both short- and long-term stays (long term is defined as over 30 days). The hospital was experiencing a significant amount of patient violence in the psychiatric wards, which was creating a fearful and dangerous work environment for the hospital staff. A staff survey revealed this to be the most important opportunity for the organization to examine with the breakthrough strategy.

PROBLEM (OPPORTUNITY) DEFINED

The first thing the hospital had to do was to identify and clearly define the performance improvement opportunity: too much violence in the psychiatric wards.

The hospital's mental health services were organized into different functions, such as nursing, psychiatry, psychology, and rehabilitation. The psychiatric wards where the patients resided were also the places where each of the functions physically came together to administer patient care. Although patient care requires coordination among the functions, typically the functions remained separate in practice. Personnel reported up their "functional silos," pursuing the aims of their function, with less emphasis on accomplishing joint objectives.

The client in this case was the director of the psychiatric wards. She polled her staff to identify improvement opportunities in the wards. The most common response, particularly from the nursing staff, was that people did not feel safe because many patients frequently acted out. In these incidents, patients would begin to lose control and become disruptive and potentially violent. These incidents could lead to patients being given sedatives or being put in restraints. If the patient did not cooperate, the staff person could be injured.

The staff made two proposals to help the situation. The first proposal was to conduct a training program for nurses on how to handle assaultive patients. The second proposal was to increase staffing levels to compensate for the high number of absent employees out on workers' compensation because of injuries resulting from patient violence.

Facilitator's Note

If the participants do not understand the problem, ask for a volunteer or pick an individual from the team and ask the rest of them to imagine what it would be like to restrain this person if he or she became disruptive and aggressive. Also ask them to imagine what it would be like if this person were six feet two inches tall and weighed 240 pounds. Ask people what they would do if they saw a patient starting to become disruptive. One response would be to look for the nearest door and let someone else deal with the situation. Another response is to ask problem-solving questions such as:

How often do these incidents occur?

What is the goal for reduction of incidents?

Who is accountable for incident reduction?

Are staffing not working together?

The answer to these questions may prompt the answers (directly) or they may begin the process of problem solving with specific quality tools (check sheets, frequency distribution, Pareto analysis, cause-and-effect diagram, brainstorming, etc.).

UNDERSTANDING THE CURRENT SITUATION

Based on the responses from the above questions and an understanding of the hierarchical structure of the hospital, the team members identified the following:

- Numerous incidents of violence every day.
- No goal for incident reduction.
- No accountability for incident reduction.
- Nurses, orderlies, psychiatrists, psychologists, and social workers not working together as effectively as possible.
- Many ideas about how to reduce violence but no plan.

Based on this understanding, a cross-functional and multidisciplinary team was formed, encompassing all staff who interacted with patients. The composition of the team was as follows:

- Head nurse (team leader).
- Two staff nurses.
- Orderly from ward.
- Clinical psychologists.
- Psychiatrist.
- Social worker.

At this stage, the team set a breakthrough goal. The team began with the opportunity and narrowed it to a razor-sharp goal. Breakthrough goals must be a measurable improvement to the existing situation and must be achievable in a matter of weeks.

Facilitator's Note

Make sure the team members understand that a training program for nurses could take many months to put together, especially if outside assistance is required. A training program also would not address many other underlying dynamics, such as the willingness of groups to collaborate and establishing accountability for reducing incidents. Training also represents a back-end fix to an upstream quality problem. If incidents could be reduced, nurses would not require training to fix them. However, by focusing on a goal of reducing incidents, the team is able to meet key criteria for a breakthrough goal: urgent and compelling, short term, measurable, and doable with existing resources and authority.

SETTING A BREAKTHROUGH GOAL

Before setting a sharp goal, the team members began problem solving by collecting data. The data they collected were directly related to the goal and served to improve their understanding of the problem. They began by examining incidents of violence that occurred during a specific month. They used a check sheet to track the following factors:

- Date and time of day.
- Patient involved.
- Location.
- Staff on duty.
- Whether sedative medication was given to bring the patient under control.
- Whether the adjustment procedure was used. (This procedure calls for isolating the patient for several minutes in a side room until the patient is able to rejoin the patient population, similar to the penalty box in ice hockey.)
- Whether the incident "snowballed" into further incidents involving other patients, who became unsettled in response to one patient acting out.

The team also collected some baseline data, with a run chart. It examined violent incidents in wards A and B for the specific month and found there were 42 incidents. The team aimed to reduce this number by 10 percent within two months, from 42 to 38 per month. The result was to streamline the original goal into the final goal in a sequence similar to the following:

From: Too much violence and injuries to staff ←————— **The opportunity**

To: Improve safety for nurses

To: Reduce levels of violence in two wards

To: Reduce incidents of violence in wards A and B by 10 percent within two months ←————— **The breakthrough goal**

At this stage, the team derived a Pareto chart from the data it collected with the check sheet and frequency distribution chart. The Pareto chart showed very clearly that patients 1 and 2 were committing a high proportion of the incidents. In Pareto terms, these patients represented the "vital few" rather than the "trivial many." This gained knowledge is very important because now the team can come up with a strategy to achieve the specified goal. The option of deinstitutionalizing the patient was not a viable option. Patient 1 had been in the hospital for two years and patient 2 for 15 months, and both still required long-term care.

TEAM FINDINGS AND ACTIONS

By collecting and analyzing data over time, the team was able to focus on a few clear findings. It took action to address these initial findings:

- Two patients are causing 45 percent of the incidents.

- Incidents tended to happen around meal time. Rather than add staff, as originally recommended, the team changed the scheduling patterns to increase coverage at meal time.

- Medication and the adjustment procedure were not being used. The team began making sure these were used as appropriate, especially with patients 1 and 2. Appropriate training (just-in-time training) was provided to achieve the goal.

- There was less snowballing of incidents due to a united staff presence. As the team began working together and collaborating more effectively, patients felt more secure due to the united staff presence. Patients had more faith that the staff would act successfully to prevent incidents or reduce the severity of the incident. Therefore, patients were less likely to act out in response to other patients.

The success that this team achieved in one month was incredible. The goal that team members had set was to reduce the number of violent incidents by 10 percent, from 44 to 38 incidents per month. In fact, they reduced the number of incidents by more than 55 percent, to just 19.

To expand the success that the team achieved, the team introduced the process to all four wards. In five months, there were 19 incidents in all wards. Based on initial levels of incidents before the team's efforts, one would have predicted more than 100 incidents across all four wards, had the improvements not been made.

TEAM RESULTS

The reduction in incidents led to a dramatic decline in staff injuries and lost workdays. The statistics are shown below:

	Before Team	After Team	% Reduction
No. of Injuries	8	2	75
Lost Workdays	144	11	92

In discussions with the original team, members indicated that another important outcome was the development of new skills, a willingness to collaborate, and confidence to tackle other challenges. The team essentially was speaking to the three aims of the breakthrough strategy, that is, new performance levels, new management skills and methods, and an increased readiness for continuous change.

At this point, the project was complete, and the team was ready to attack a new problem.

CHAPTER 14

Customer Service

This chapter addresses the issue of customer service. Specifically, it recognizes the need for customer service and attempts to explain the concept from a futuristic perspective. In the process, customer service is examined thoroughly, and the rationale is provided based on the assumption that customer service in healthcare is not a competitive advantage; rather, it is the price of doing business.

As customer service emerges as a competitive imperative during the next decade, organizations that anticipate the power of information technology and employ it creatively in their service infrastructures should enjoy a distinct competitive advantage over their rivals. To be successful in the 1990s and beyond, companies must recognize and deal with the convergence of two indisputable forces: the primacy of customer service as a competitive weapon and the pervasive role of information technology in the value chain. These are not independent forces. Although information technology (IT) has the ability to redefine businesses, alter industry structure, and foster entirely new types of enterprise, its greatest unrealized potential is in the area of customer service.

CUSTOMER SERVICE DEFINED

The concept of high-quality customer service is difficult to define, especially in healthcare. Everyone seems to recognize quality service when they experience it. However, defining customer service that is perceived as high quality is complicated because it involves individual perceptions.

Healthcare customers typically do not merely regard the finished product as the measure of service but will also take into account the process by which the finished product was obtained, the overall experience. This may include the time it takes to obtain the service, the friendliness of the medical staff, and so on. An outstanding performance on one aspect can help overcome a mediocre performance on another.

Another factor that complicates the evaluation of quality customer service is that the only opinion or point of view that matters is that of the customer. Customer service may meet all the criteria for quality, but if, according to the customer, it is lacking some key ingredient, then it fails as quality customer service. Therefore, service quality, as perceived by customers, can be defined as the extent of discrepancy between customers' expectations or desires and their perceptions.

The next key factor is to determine which criteria define the customers' expectations of quality service. The Marketing Science Institute of Cambridge, Massachusetts, identified 10 dimensions of service quality in focus group studies. These dimensions are as follows: tangibles, reliability, responsiveness, competence, courtesy, credibility, security, access, communication, and understanding the customer. For a detailed explanation of these items, see Zeithaml, Parasuraman, and Berry (1990). These 10 dimensions, to varying degrees, are consciously or subconsciously used by the customer to assess the quality level or the service received. The customer then compares the assessed level to his or her preconceived expectations. Shortfalls result in customer dissatisfaction.

Almost all organizations compete on service to some degree. Does the Cleveland Clinic sell open heart surgeries or the personal attention, expertise, and overall care that comes with and after the surgery? The perceived quality of all processes involved in the purchase and service experience balanced against expectations determines whether the customer will return to the clinic.

There are several factors contributing to organizations' emphasis on quality customer service that will accelerate and become more acute in the years to come. For example, in the early 1980s, U.S. customers, largely as a result of Japanese product and service quality, began to demand high-quality products and services.

Manufacturers in the United States responded by refocusing their attention on product quality and by redesigning their manufacturing processes. In the late 1980s many industries (service and manufacturing) noted that customer service provides a distinct competitive advantage. Companies began to realize that in many cases, growth was not due to technological breakthroughs, but service breakthroughs. These organizations also realized that the growth leaders in their industries were also service leaders.

Technological enhancements to existing products as well as the proliferation of products and services create customer confusion and the subsequent need for additional sales service. As the pace of technological change accelerates, customer service will increase in value as a competitive advantage. Naisbitt (1989, p. 19) has noted that the more high tech the world becomes, the more people crave high touch. Personalized service that takes into account the needs of the individual will play a major role in future service trends. Organizations, however, must be careful not to fall into the trap of serving a few customers very well and the majority poorly.

According to the U.S. Office of Consumer Affairs, 90 percent of dissatisfied customers will not buy again (Daniel 1992). Moreover, Stamatis (Technial Assistance Research Programs, White House Office of Consumer Affairs, 1995) reports that a dissatisfied customer will tell at least nine other people of the unpleasant experience. The multiplier effect indicates that it would not be long before quality-conscious customers purchase elsewhere.

One will agree that the ultimate reason for quality customer service is the bottom line. In the short run, however, it is difficult to point out the effects of quality service on the bottom-line since it is a long-term business strategy. When bottom line accounting management rules organizations, cutting costs can undermine service to the customer.

Over the long term, the most profitable organizations have delivered strong customer service. It has been consistently shown that the consumer will pay a premium for quality customer service. If an organization does not deliver high-quality service, its product or service becomes a commodity and thereby commands only commodity prices. Most organizations are pretty competitive on price. However, only one product or service can have the lowest price. Service is the number one factor for differentiation.

How do we involve the coming technological change into enhancing healthcare service? First and foremost we need to set our priorities. In the past, healthcare organizations looked for and relied on major technological breakthroughs to help improve productivity and quality. In the future, the same organizations will also need to look for technology to improve customer service. As Kahn (1991, p. 56) points out, there is a big difference between maximizing technology for improved customer service and maximizing customer service through technology. Never conclude that technology is a direct route to improved customer service.

CUSTOMER SERVICE TECHNOLOGIES

Today the use of technologies in business to improve productivity, quality, and customer service is changing rapidly. Although many organizations are still using outdated mainframe information systems, some organizations are leapfrogging the competition by using more advanced, integrated information systems enhanced by recently developed technologies such as electronic data interchange (EDI), cellular phones, and compact disk–read only memory. Specific applications follow.

Relational Database Management Systems (RDBMS)

RDBMS systems store large amounts of related data in fields. The advantage of the system is the speed with which the information can be manipulated and accessed. Hundreds of fields of information for a given topic can be stored and the user can selectively retrieve the information that is pertinent at that time. Since the RDBMS systems are on-line, data requests can easily be duplicated, thereby eliminating the need to refile the information and, with it, the waste associated with redundant data.

Good examples of effective uses in healthcare of RDBMS systems are admissions, medical records, and the customer processing system. The benefit from having an integrated system is the ability to have immediate information regarding the customer and/or the system. Another way that healthcare can use this system is by providing customer service to their customers and the community on an on-line access to product and service databases.

The customer calls into an 800 number and through a series of query screens is given information about the organization's products and services.

Addressability/Databased Marketing

Addressability or databased marketing uses database technology to allow organizations to track customer preferences and tailor promotion and advertising to specific customer needs. In healthcare this may be used in reminding customers of upcoming tests and new programs that the customers may have identified that they are interested in.

Another aspect of this addressability and database technology is the compact disk–read only memory. This technology allows the storage of data on a 4.75-inch optical disk for information retrieval. In healthcare this can be used to convert documents (e.g., imaging records) into computerized data. Another application may be to use the system in such a way that numerous people simultaneously access medical records and information.

Multimedia

Multimedia technology uses the personal computer and combines it with audio, video, text, graphics, and animation. The applications are limitless. They depend on the availability of phone equipment, which can effectively transmit the massive amounts of data required to support the system. Applications in healthcare include the use of multimedia for customers to better understand the organization's goals and services. Multimedia also can be used internally to explain in a friendly mode the organization's pension plan as well as provide training programs and user manuals to supplement conventional training programs.

Electronic Data Interchange

EDI has become a necessity in recent years in business-to-business communication. It has resulted in a significant improvement in accuracy and reliability of customer service. In healthcare this system can be used in billing the direct customer (patients) as well as billing third-party institutions (insurance, Medicaid/Medicare, etc.).

Other Technologies

The use of local area networks (LANs), computers with modems, the Internet, cellular phones, fax machines, and electronic mail is increasing in a geometric fashion. All of these technologies may be used to increase the level of customer service, provided that they are not thought of as new approaches to customer service but rather tools for a more effective approach to communication.

STATE-OF-THE ART TECHNOLOGIES

Virtual Reality

Some Japanese organizations are already experimenting with the use of virtual reality technology, whereby a customer can actually experience the product or service. Virtual reality is a highly sophisticated simulation software that allows customers to choose, change, and participate in the environment of their choice. Although the possibilities of this technology are potentially endless, they are extremely costly.

Expert Systems

Expert systems are electronic decision trees that enable a less experienced user to use information files for product and process design or diagnostics. These decision trees allow complex jobs normally requiring highly specialized individuals to be handled by office personnel with rudimentary computer skills. Another area that organizations are investing in is after-the-service information systems. In healthcare, expert systems may be used for poison control advice, first-aid diagnostics, and as a troubleshooting checklist.

Artificial Intelligence

While real-time information accessibility and availability are the building blocks of information systems in the future, development of sophisticated decision support systems using artificial intelligence technology will be the basis for running the high-velocity businesses of the future. Constantly changing market conditions will reduce businesses' ability to recoup product investment costs as product life cycles decline. The complexity of daily and long-term business decisions will increase to the point where use of artificial intelligence and expert information systems will be mandatory for survival. The complex algorithms developed for the advanced systems will have to be monitored carefully and adjusted to avoid obsolescence.

MANAGEMENT OF TECHNOLOGY

With these technologies, one of the key issues is the type of organizational form that the organization of the future will take. There certainly will be a representation from all types of corporate hierarchies, but because of the dynamics of the information age, we believe the popular organizational form—especially in healthcare—will be an "adhocracy." This type of organization, in which a core group forms management teams to complete certain projects and then disbands the teams, seems particularly suited to the types of technology of the future. As one has the ability to connect with various groups and individuals using computer messages, fax machines, and eventually video telephones, it is no longer necessary to form project groups in the same city or even the same country. This concept appears congruent with an adhocracy organization, which attempts to capture a floating pool of talent for the project at hand and then moves on and uses the next group of experts for the following project. In the increasing global economy, technological communications will be critical to linking the various elements of the organization together.

One trend that is prevalent and expanding is the use of outsourcing. As technology becomes more complex and greater expertise is needed to handle information systems and technology, it will become too expensive for organizations to maintain quality staffs in-house. Therefore, an acceleration in outsourcing contracts for maintenance and upgrades of information systems will be required. This process is really just an early form of an adhocracy.

The key element to enhancing quality customer service in the future through technology is a concept called reengineering the work flow. The essence of reengineering is for management to challenge the status quo for all work flow and to redesign it to fit the available technology. For more details, see Stamatis (1996), Manganelli and Klein (1994), and Hammer and Champy (1993).

What do these technologies have to do with customer service, and how does an organization's management go about implementing technology to improve customer service? As with all changes, and especially with customer service, the changes must occur at the top. Top management must have a vision and develop a strategic plan to implement quality customer service. For the mechanics of implementing total quality service, see Stamatis (1995). To accomplish this, the system must be designed in such a way that optimal flexibility at the customer contact point is achieved. Also, maximum production efficiencies from constant repetition, experience-curve effects, and cost quality control must be obtained.

A redesign of the system should increase efficiency and also empower the front-line employees. This is a critical facet in improving and maintaining quality customer service and achieving improvement in efficiency. Properly designed service technology systems allow relatively inexperienced people to perform very sophisticated tasks, quickly vaulting them over normal learning curve delays. By constant updating, the most successful technologies and systems automatically capture the highest potential experience curve benefits available in the entire system. This allows employees to take advantage of the total organization's constantly expanding capabilities, which they could not possibly learn firsthand or be trained to execute personally. This is also the most difficult managerial act because it involves giving up control and power, which managers have always craved. The key here is control. Empower the front-line people with the ability to satisfy the customer and have management systems via technology in place to monitor and inform the employees of mistakes.

An organizational design intended to facilitate the ability of the front-line personnel is an inverted organization, whereby all support systems and managers exist to help personnel with customer contact serve the customer. This properly places the focus where it should be—on the customer.

Another advantage that technology provides is that it can create a flat organization. With properly implemented technological systems, the number of people reporting to one individual can be increased dramatically. Some maintain that an infinite number can report to one individual, but technology does have its limits. Nonetheless, many layers of management or individual managers can be eliminated for efficiency and bottom-line improvement. As more effective software is brought on board, an infinitely flat organization is theoretically possible by a rules-based central control system. Whether that would be desirable for customer service remains to be seen.

To achieve the empowerment of the front-line worker, extensive training and retraining are necessary. The skills employees have today are rapidly becoming obsolete as technological change rolls on. The sooner an organization implements extensive training programs, the less the organization will have to catch up in the future. Change both inside and outside of the organization is embedded in the future. The better that employees understand and cope with change, the faster they will evolve with the technology.

REFERENCES

Daniel, A. L. "Overcome the Barriers to Superior Customer Service." *Journal of Business Strategy*, January/February 1992, pp. 18–24.

Hammer, M., and J. Champy. *Reengineering the Corporation*. New York: Harper Business, 1993.

Kahn, A. "Maximize Customer Service through Technology." *Chain Store Age Executive*, October 1991, p. 56.

Manganelli, R. L., and M. M. Klein. *The Reengineering Handbook*. New York: AMACOM, 1994.

Naisbitt, J. "Megatrends: Ten New Directions Transforming Our Lives." In *Total Customer Service*. W. H. Davidow and B. Uttal, eds. New York: Harper & Row, 1989.

Stamatis, D. H. *Total Quality Service*. Delray Beach, Fla.: St. Lucie Press, 1995.

———. *Creating the Future: The Nuts and Bolts of Reengineering*. Red Bluff, Calif.: Paton Press, 1996.

Zeithaml, V. A.; A. Parasuraman; and L. L. Berry. *Delivering Quality Service*. New York: Free Press, 1990.

Deming's Updated 14 Points

The following 14 points are the updated version of the original 14 obligations of top management. These points are based on a video narrated by Lloyd Dobyns and part of the Deming Library Series. In volume 16, *The Quality Leader,* Dobyns attributes these new updates to Dr. W. Edwards Deming. The updated points and the original versions are listed here.

1. Create and publish to all employees a statement of the aims and purposes of the company or other organization. The management must demonstrate constantly its commitment to this statement.
   Old: Create constancy of purpose for service improvement.
2. Learn the new philosophy (top management and everybody).
   Old: Adopt the new philosophy.
3. Understand the purpose of inspection for improvement of processes and reduction of cost.
   Old: Cease dependence on inspection to achieve quality.
4. End the practice of awarding business on the basis of price tag alone.
   Old: End the practice of awarding business on price alone; make partners out of vendors.
5. Improve constantly and forever the system of production and service.
   Old: Constantly improve every process for planning, production, and service.
6. Institute training.
   Old: Institute training and retraining on the job.
7. Teach and institute leadership.
   Old: Institute leadership for system improvement.
8. Drive out fear. Create trust. Create a climate for innovation.
   Old: Drive out fear.

9. Optimize toward the aims and purposes of the company the efforts of teams, groups, and staff areas.

   Old: Break down barriers between staff areas.

10. Eliminate exhortations for the workforce.

    Old: Eliminate slogans, exhortations, and targets for the workforce.

11a. Eliminate numerical quotas for production. Instead learn and institute methods for improvement.

11b. Eliminate MBO (management by objectives). Instead, learn the capabilities of processes and how to improve them.

    Old: Eliminate numerical quotas for the workforce and numerical goals for the management.

12. Remove barriers that rob people of pride of workmanship.

    Old: Remove barriers to pride of workmanship.

13. Encourage education and self-improvement for everyone.

    Old: Institute a vigorous program of education and self-improvement for everyone.

14. Take action to accomplish the transformation.

    Old: Put everyone to work on the transformation.

Goals and Their Development

To be effective, a team needs to know where it is going. Selection of an improvement goal or theme provides focus and direction for the team's problem-solving efforts. A famous quotation from *Alice in Wonderland* makes the point.

> *Alice:* Which way do I go from here?
>
> *Cat:* That depends on where you want to go.
>
> *Alice:* I don't know where I'm going.
>
> *Cat:* Then it doesn't matter which way you go.

PURPOSES OF GOAL SETTING

An improvement goal strengthens team performance in three ways. First, a goal provides focus for the team's activities. All the problems of an organization can't be addressed simultaneously. A goal provides focus for problem solving.

A goal also provides a framework for achievement motivation. It is hard to get a sense of satisfaction from your efforts without a specific target or goal for which to reach. Without a target, you will never know whether you are improving.

Finally, a goal provides a way for the team to evaluate its problem-solving activities. If the team sets an improvement goal and then attacks the problems related to that goal, it should be able to see tangible progress. Only with a goal and a feedback system can a team assess its impact on the organization.

TECHNIQUES FOR SETTING IMPROVEMENT GOALS AND ESTABLISHING FEEDBACK

Characteristics of Improvement Goals

A good team improvement goal should have the following characteristics:

> *Results oriented*—The goal should be set in a specific area of the group's performance (i.e., focused on achieving results).

Measurable—The result area selected for a goal should be as measurable as possible.

Challenging but reasonable—The goal should require a stretch beyond current performance but should be attainable.

Clearly understood—The goal should be viewed as a meaningful measure of the group's performance.

Controllable—The group should be able to impact the goal area through its efforts. Avoid goals that are heavily influenced by external factors.

Posted—Public display of the goal strengthens commitment.

Establishing Feedback

Setting the goal establishes the improvement target. A feedback system is needed to help the team assess its progress toward the goal. Feedback allows the team to take greater responsibility for its own progress. A feedback system should provide information that is specific, timely, understandable, and clearly related to the goal.

Team members should be involved in measuring progress and posting the results. The best technique for tracking progress is a control chart. A control chart is a method for a team to track progress on a goal or to evaluate the effect of an implemented solution.

Behaviors to Help a Team Set an Improvement Goal

The team leader should do the following:

1. Discuss the value of goal setting and focus the team on (possible) result areas.

2. Review organizational trends, goals, results, or problem areas. Share with the team any data that could shed light on the team's performance and indicate possible areas for improvement.

3. Ask the group to identify possible goal areas. After sharing the relevant information, solicit ideas for possible goals.

4. Have the team select the goal or theme. Through discussion and perhaps ranking, have the team select a goal. It is important to make this a team decision to ensure commitment.

5. Specify the goal. Once the goal has been selected, try to

specify the goals in terms of measures, time period, and amount of improvement.

Skills in Goal Setting

Use the following techniques for team goal setting:

1. Make goal statements descriptive and concise:

   The more abstract the language, the less precise the goal.

   The less precise the goal, the slimmer the chances of accomplishing it.

   Ambiguity leads to tangents, confusion, and more ambiguity.

   Descriptiveness leads to operational and behavioral goals.

   Descriptiveness allows to you to reach consensus on measuring a goal.

2. Make goal statements complete:

   Determine that operations will allow you to accomplish the task.

   Include behavioral, performance-based data.

   Establish that the goal is suitable, doable, and reachable.

3. Make goal statements consistent:

   Differentiate between personal and group goals.

   Compare short-term and long-term goals.

   Make sure goals can be accomplished in the given time limit.

4. Make members accountable:

   Use subgoals and realistic deadlines.

   Describe expectations verbally and in writing.

   Establish feedback procedures.

SUMMARY OF GOAL SETTING

Objective

- To establish a specific improvement goal to focus the group's efforts.

Pitfalls

- Lack of focus.
- Vague reasons for meetings.
- No boundaries.
- Unable to assess impact of problem solving.

Useful Technique

- Review control data.

Leader Emphasis

- Share information on goals, results, trends, and broader problems.
- Establish guidelines.
- Solicit goal ideas.
- Specify goals.
- Seek commitment from team members.

What Would You Do If . . . ?
Troubleshooting

This appendix is designed to provide the reader with some troubleshooting ideas in the process of implementing the TQM breakthrough strategy in an organization. It is not an exhaustive analysis; however, it provides some of the most frequent problems and solutions that a facilitator can implement.

COMMON PROBLEMS

Team Wants to Change Goal

Particularly in the first few weeks, a team will often feel overwhelmed by the tasks and training, experience major obstacles early on, and generally feel overchallenged about the expected work. Since change usually provokes anxieties, it is important for a facilitator to listen to and acknowledge particular feelings but to also urge the team to keep trying because this is a typical part of the breakthrough process. The purpose of the goal is to hold everyone to the same course, which helps get change actually happening. Any change to the goal will not keep that necessary pressure on.

Of course, if in looking at the preliminary baseline data, it is obvious that the team did not understand what it was taking on, there could be a slight adjustment. And if the sponsor feels that the goal is not significant enough, you may want to have that individual discuss increasing the goal with the team or the team leader.

Team Leader Thinks Goal
Will Be Achieved Late

The team leader may ask for time extensions. Unless there are extenuating circumstances, the answer is *no!* Time deadlines help push change. Otherwise, actions necessary for today's deadline will be put off until tomorrow.

Teams Runs into Early Obstacle

One thing that breakthrough projects show very early is how "normal" absence, sickness, new workloads, changes, and so on are actually part of "typical" days. Obviously, some obstacles are more unusual and uncontrollable than others, but typically all obstacles are initially experienced as insurmountable. It is important that these ongoing business realities not be used as an excuse for inability to do a project or reach a goal.

Obviously, if one critical person on the team becomes seriously ill or some major new system is being implemented or there is some similar major obstacle, there is cause for rethinking the project. However, keep the stages of the breakthrough team dynamics in mind; in the first few weeks, teams will feel uncertain, doubtful, overwhelmed, and naturally will be looking for ways (obstacles) to take away some anxiety. Your role as facilitator is to help first the team leader and second the sponsor assess the extent and nature of the obstacles, and take appropriate actions.

Team Does Not Seem to Own the Goal

Your role is to try to understand why and help the team leader and/or sponsor overcome this barrier. Look at issues such as:

- Does the team feel that the opportunity is important?
- Has the sponsor been clear enough with the demand?
- Are team members unmotivated for other reasons?
- Has something not been addressed that has become an obstacle to achieving the goal?
- Has the team leader taken on too much or too little?

Facilitator Feels Success of Project Depends on Him or Her

As a general guideline, the team needs you as their primary supporter, not as an active participant on their work plan. If the team does ask you to take on an action step, make sure they know that you are supposed to act as a facilitator and ask if anyone could take on that action step and come to you as a source of information. If your team is sure that only you can take on that step, consider whether that step is absolutely necessary before you take it on.

Team Is Not Achieving Goal

One of your key responsibilities is to help keep the team focused on the goal. If the team has completed its action steps but is not achieving the goal, help them ask questions such as:

- Were the original action steps in the work plan inadequate?
- Were the action steps completed well and properly?
- Is there a particular obstacle that has been encountered that needs a higher level of intervention that the team could request?
- Is the team pushing hard enough?
- Is the project too dependent on one person or action as the major factor in achieving the goal?
- Last resort: Is the goal too big and/or too much of a stretch?

Team Has Trouble Gaining Cooperation outside the Team

As part of your support role, you can help the team consider what to do if it has trouble gaining cooperation from departments not represented on the team. Ask:

- Should the team consider adding someone from the uncooperative group?
- Has the team shared compelling factual data with this group?
- Has the team considered how it would be in that group's self-interest to cooperate? If there is no self-interest, has the team considered other incentives to gain cooperation?

As a last resort, have the team leader seek higher authority (from a sponsor or senior manager) to gain the necessary push for cooperation.

Sponsor Is Not Playing His or Her Part

The sponsor must balance a hands-off approach of letting the team take charge while showing interest, giving support, and intervening only when it becomes necessary. If you see an imbalance of either overinvolvement or underinvolvement, the question is how to address this with the sponsor. In this case, it will depend on your relationship, both formal (position) and informal (personal), with the sponsor.

It is important to have the team try to get the necessary level of involvement without assistance. However, if it is appropriate only for you to say or to do something, try to stay focused on the goal and discuss how certain things won't be able to happen if the sponsor acts or does not act. Periodically ask the sponsor how he or she thinks the project is going. The main emphasis for you is to help the team get what it needs to achieve the goal. The more the team members can get what they need for themselves, the stronger and more empowered they will be in the end.

Team Oversteps Its Role

Sometimes a team feels so "empowered" that it makes decisions and takes actions that supersede its authority. Perhaps it is time for a new definition of what role is appropriate; sometimes it takes experimenting with a new way to see if it works. However, if the team has taken on too much, it is usually the role of a sponsor or senior manager to draw the line. Try to have this person praise the team for trying out something new but gently be firm about the consequences of their actions. Finally, one way this can be avoided is for the team to put an experimental action step on the work plan; when the sponsor and senior manager review the work plan, they can give feedback before anything inappropriate happens.

Personnel Issues Hinder Goal Achievement

If one or more team members are causing problems and are affecting the team's ability to achieve the goal, consider the following:

- Raise these issues with the team leader; discuss whether to consider them with the individual or team.

- Help the team leader figure out whether to ask the senior manager or sponsor to step in.
- Give the problematic person or persons a chance to change; breakthrough projects can elicit new behaviors and attitudes.

As a last resort, speak with the sponsor. Realize, however, that the sponsor may raise the issue in a way that you might not agree with, so think through the possibilities beforehand.

Team Members Feel They Have Too Much to Do

First, it may be true that the team members have too much to do. If so, consider that this may not be the right time for a breakthrough with this particular team; discuss this with the sponsor and set up a commitment with the team as to when will be a better time for them to take on the opportunity. Second, in most cases, there is extra work at the beginning of the project, and many members may feel stretched. It might be helpful for you to confirm this as part of the process and give examples of how other breakthrough projects were worth this short-term additional time investment.

Team Leader Is Doing Too Much or Too Little

A team leader guides, coordinates, motivates, and takes on action steps. If the team leader is doing all the work, what kind of ownership will team members feel? If that individual takes on too little, will the team feel dumped on, as if the team is not a priority for the team leader? Point out the consequences to the team leader. If he or she takes on too much work, the team may not take on responsibility for changes. If the leader takes on too little, the team may not see the project as a priority.

Team Leader Avoids You

Sometimes a team leader does not return phone calls and resists meeting with you. The best approach is to be direct and ask team leader why. As a last resort, discuss the leader's conduct with the sponsor.

Facilitator Is Manager of the Team Leader

If the team leader reports directly to you, consider the following options:

- It could be useful to learn to incorporate facilitating into your management style; since you are used to managing this person, focus on facilitating.
- If there is another facilitator, switch teams.

Training for Breakthrough Strategy in Healthcare

This appendix provides a typical training program for implementing the TQM–breakthrough strategy in a healthcare work environment. Two examples are given: one hospital and one HMO. In the case of the hospital, I provide the sequence for training, covering the basic concepts of total quality management and the basic tools. For the HMO, I provide the organization's outline for improvement (stated in seven steps) and its sequence of analysis. For a more detailed approach to TQM implementation and training curriculum, see D. H. Stamatis, *Total Quality Service* (Delray Beach, Fla.: St. Lucie Press, 1995).

TQM TRAINING IN A HOSPITAL

Objectives:

1. To introduce an organization leadership group to the theory of TQM and the role of a quality council within TQM.

2. To provide opportunities for the quality council to form as a team within a quality framework.

3. To provide a quality council with the information it needs to oversee and implement quality improvement (QI) projects.

4. To introduce the concepts of quality planning to the organization.

The first of seven sessions teaches the following tools and topics:

Tools Taught	Topics
Brainstorming	Overview of TQM philosophy and breakthrough strategy and its role in organization; roles of quality council
Nominal group technique, multiple voting	Brief overview of history and benefits of TQM in healthcare; introduction to principles of quality: ■ Process thinking ■ Customer and suppliers ■ Cost of quality ■ Variation ■ Continuous quality improvement (CQI)
Meeting management skills	

The outcome of this session should be that the team develops criteria for selecting the hospital's pilot QI projects.

The second session teaches the following:

Tools Taught	Topics
Flowcharts	The place of divergent and convergent thinking in QI projects
Cause-and-effect diagram	Why QI projects use tools, and what kind of tools are used where; specific information on tools for process description
Data collection tools	What quality councils should know before teams collect data

The outcomes for the training groups should be as follows:

■ Hands-on experience in constructing flowcharts from team dialogue and understanding how this skill would be useful to a quality council.

■ Hands-on experience in creating a data collection plan from a team dialogue case study.

In session 3, the group learns the following:

Tools Taught	Topics
Pareto diagram	Pareto principle (vital as opposed to trivial): how to get the most payoff for your QI effort
Histogram	Patterns of variation: what they tell us about how processes are working
Control charts	Special-cause and common-cause variation: understanding what this concept means for management

The outcome of the third session should be creation of problem statements and selection of QI teams from a case study of medication error data.

Session 4:

Tools Taught	Topics
Review of QI tools	Case study, which takes team through simulated QI project from beginning to end

The outcome should be an understanding, through hands-on experience, of how the CQI process actually works.

Session 5:

Tools Taught	Topics
Brainstorming (refresher)	What is a good problem statement?
Multivoting (refresher)	What direction the quality council should give a team; what belongs in a team's mission statement

The outcome should be a preliminary list generated by the team of possibilities for that organization's pilot QI project or projects.

Session 6:

Tools Taught	Topics
Multivoting (refresher continued)	Review of originally selected criteria
Consensus	Changes or additions
Use of matrixes for decision making	Evaluation of possible projects against chosen criteria

As the outcome, the team should prepare one or two pilot quality improvement projects with mission statements.

Session 7 teaches the following:

Tools Taught	Topics
Affinity diagrams and affinity process	Back to TQM and the importance of quality planning
Process	Examples of other hospitals' implementation plans
Interrelationship diagrams	Introduction to some advanced quality tools

Outcome: As a result of hands-on experience of working through how an affinity process diagram actually works, the team should understand key next steps in continuing CQI and TQM efforts at this hospital.

HMO DEFINITION AND IMPLEMENTATION OF THE BREAKTHROUGH STRATEGY

Step	Objective
1. Reason for improvement	Identify problem (opportunity) and reason for working on it
2. Current situation	Select a problem and set a target for improvement; team collects and interprets data to help key in on one project
3. Analysis	Show the team's identification and verification of root causes of problem (rather than symptoms of problem) before proceeding to next step; team brainstorms, conducts cause-and-effect analysis (e.g., fishbone diagram, scatter plot diagram) and identifies root causes through use of Pareto diagram, histogram, etc.
	Once problem has been isolated, team moves into higher order tools—if applicable—to determine variation, capability, and stability of process generating problem.
4. Action for improvement	Show action for improvement (proposed solutions) selected by team that will correct identified root causes of problem. Typical approaches are:
	a. Develop action for improvement matrix
	▪ Problem
	▪ Root cause
	▪ Actions
	▪ Practical methods
	▪ Barriers
	▪ Aids, i.e., storyboard, flowchart
	b. Perform cost analysis
	c. Action plan
5. Results	Confirm that problem and its root causes have been decreased and target for improvement has been met; make preliminary preparations for presentation
6. Follow-up	Prevent problem and its root causes from recurring; once data in results section indicate that actions for improvement have been successful, team begins to standardize its system for improvement. (This may be accomplished with a variety of charts, standards, or procedures that are used to monitor process activity and that maintain emphasis on reducing variation.)
7. Future plans	Allow team a chance to review its story and address any remaining issues

Lessons Learned

This appendix provides the reader with some lessons I have learned over the years in trying to implement total quality management.

Lesson 1. Invest in TQM only if the executive team is personally willing to make a convincing case for change. Employees work harder when they know the administration (executive team) can provide a compelling vision that gives TQM meaning and purpose.

Lesson 2. Enlist 100 percent support from physicians and middle managers. Give them leading roles in the TQM process.

Lesson 3. Align organization incentives to reinforce TQM objectives. Revise job descriptions, performance evaluations, and compensation systems to ensure that the staff receives consistent signals regarding the priority of TQM initiatives.

Lesson 4. Develop a long-term strategy and use it to drive TQM. Without perspective of what it will take to succeed over the long run, TQM efforts are just a shot in the dark.

Lesson 5. Prioritize TQM efforts, focusing first and foremost on the most important customer groups. For most healthcare organizations, this will mean physicians and payers. The implication is that top-priority objectives will be low-cost, efficient healthcare delivery and unquestionable clinical quality rather than patient satisfaction. To set priorities, we recommend the following steps:

1. Does the project address the needs of the healthcare organization's top-priority customer group?

2. Does the project address important needs of the customer, which can have an impact on the customer's selection decision for a provider?

3. Is the healthcare organization far ahead of the competition in this area already (i.e., will improvement have any effect on the bottom line)?

4. Does this project truly offer the organization a good chance of making an improvement large enough to change customer behavior?

5. Will the project require an investment large enough to wipe out any potential gain?
6. How does the project rank on the preceding criteria in relation to other possible projects?
7. Once the project is selected, is the team continuously assessing whether the project is the best one to move the department and the organization toward their goals?

Lesson 6. Do not become a slave to orthodoxy over empiricism. Many healthcare organizations are rigidly adhering to TQM doctrine without consideration of what is working and what is not. For example: an organization may go overboard on employee empowerment to the point where the decision making of the management is hindered. In the same vein, do not become dogmatic on which quality philosophy (e.g., Deming, Crosby, or Juran) to follow.

Lesson 7. Hold TQM accountable to the bottom line. It is absolutely legitimate to set cost reduction and profit improvement goals within the TQM scope.

Lesson 8. Set aggressive goals for every team and every department; however, make sure they are attainable and realistic for the time allotted. Hold people accountable for achieving goals, not only for participation in the TQM process but also for substantive results.

Lesson 9. Accelerate the process and maintain momentum. Many healthcare organizations send signals that they are in no hurry for results, laying out a four- or five-year plan for project completion and a six- to eight-year plan for big results on their investment. Going slowly can have disastrous effects of sapping motivation and compromising outcome. Without a belief in urgency of the mission, employee commitment to TQM at best is half-hearted.

Lesson 10. Compress the time taken to get TQM off the ground. Avoid delays, which sap organizational energy and enthusiasm for change, by jump-starting TQM with streamlined training and a perfect pilot program.

Lesson 11. Focus tightly on the TQM effort. Concentrating organizational energies on a handful of issues ensures that project results will build on each other to produce noticeable change and true competitive advantage.

Lesson 12. Do not waste time reinventing the wheel. Benchmark processes against the best of the best to expand teams' thinking, stimulate creative solutions, and leverage results. Benchmarking can be conducted with other healthcare organizations and with organizations outside healthcare.

Lesson 13. Increase team efficiency. Set realistic deadlines, and help teams meet them by clearly defining the focus of the project and by offering the help of consultants for data collection and analysis.

Lesson 14. Make sure results stick. Management must institute measurement and control systems to ensure that improvements are maintained.

Formulas Used
in Quality Management

This appendix provides some typical formulas used in the quality profession. The list is by no means exhaustive; however, it provides the quality professional with some basic approaches to statistical understanding for the everyday application of quality management to real problems. Part I provides the most common formulas, and Part II provides the formulas for calculating control chart limits and capability. Part III provides the appropriate constants used in the provided formulas.

I. GENERAL FORMULAS

1. Arithmetic mean (average) from ungrouped data

For a population:

$$\mu = \frac{\sum X}{N}$$

For a sample:

$$\bar{X} = \frac{\sum X}{n}$$

For the average of the average:

$$\bar{\bar{X}} = \frac{\sum \bar{X}}{n}$$

where

$\sum X$ = Sum of all observed population (or sample) values
N = Number of observations in the population
n = Number of observations in the sample
$\sum \bar{X}$ = Average of the samples

2. Arithmetic mean (average) from grouped data

For a population:

$$\mu = \frac{\sum fX}{N}$$

For a sample:

$$\bar{X} = \frac{\sum fX}{n}$$

where

$\sum fX$ = Sum of all class frequency (f) times class midpoint (X) products

N = Number of observations in the population

n = Number of observations in the sample

3. Median from ungrouped data

For a population:

$$M = X_{\frac{N+1}{2}} \text{ in an ascending ordered array}$$

For a sample:

$$m = X_{\frac{n+1}{2}} \text{ in an ascending ordered array}$$

where

X = Observed population (or sample) value

N = Number of observations in the population

n = Number of observations in the sample

4. Median from grouped data

For a population:

$$M = L + \frac{\left(n/2\right) - F}{f} w$$

For a sample:

$$m = L + \frac{\left(n/2\right) - F}{f} w$$

where

L = Lower limit of median class

f = Absolute frequency of median class

w = Width of median class

F = Sum of frequencies up to (but not including) the median class

N = Number of observations in the population

n = Number of observations in the sample

5. Mode from grouped data

For a population or a sample:

$$MO \text{ or } mo = L + \frac{d_1}{d_1 + d_2}\, w$$

where

L = Lower limit of modal class

w = Width of modal class

d_1 = Difference between modal class frequency density and that of the preceding class

d_2 = Difference between modal class frequency density and that of the following class

6. Weighted mean from ungrouped data

For a population:

$$\mu_w = \frac{\sum wX}{\sum w}$$

For a sample:

$$\bar{x}_w = \frac{\sum wX}{\sum w}$$

where

$\sum w_1 X$ = Sum of all weight (w) times observed-value (x) products

$\sum w$ = N (number of observations in the population) or n (number of observations in the sample)

7. Mean absolute deviation

From ungrouped data:

For a population:

$$MAD = \frac{\sum |X - \mu|}{N}$$

For a sample:

$$MAD = \frac{\sum |X - \bar{X}|}{n}$$

where

$\sum |X - \mu|$ = Sum of the absolute differences between each
observed population value, X, and the
population mean, μ

N = Number of observations in the population

$\sum |X - \bar{x}|$ = Sum of the absolute differences between each
observed sample value, X, and the sample
mean, $\bar{X}$

n = Number of observations in the sample

From grouped data:

Denoting absolute class frequencies by f and class midpoints by X, substitute $\sum f |X - \mu|$ or $\sum f |X - \bar{X}|$ for the numerators given here.

Note: Occasionally absolute deviations from the median rather than from the mean are calculated, in which case μ is replaced by M, and $\bar{X}$ is replaced by m.

8. Variance from ungrouped data

For a population:

$$\sigma^2 \frac{\sum (x - \mu)^2}{N}$$

For a sample:

$$s^2 \frac{\sum (x - \bar{x})^2}{n - 1}$$

where

$\sum (x - \mu)^2$ = Sum of squared deviations between each
population value, X, and the population mean,
μ

N = Number of observations in the population

$\sum (x - \bar{x})^2$ = Sum of squared deviations between each sample value, X, and the sample mean, $\bar{x}$

n = Number of observations in the sample

9. Variance from grouped data

For a population:

$$\sigma^2 \frac{\sum f(x - \mu)^2}{N}$$

For a sample:

$$s^2 \frac{\sum f(x - \bar{x})^2}{n - 1}$$

where

f = Absolute class frequencies
x = Class midpoints of grouped population (or sample) values
μ = Population
$\bar{x}$ = Sample
N = Number of observations in the population
n = Number of observations in the sample

10. Standard deviation from ungrouped data

For a population:

$$\sigma = \sqrt{\frac{\sum (x - \mu)^2}{N}}$$

For a sample:

$$s = \sqrt{\frac{\sum (x - \bar{x})^2}{n - 1}}$$

where

$\sum (x - \mu)^2$ = Sum of squared deviations between each population value, x, and the population mean, μ

N = Number of observations in the population

$\sum (x - \bar{x})^2$ = Sum of squared deviations between each sample value, x, and the sample mean, $\bar{x}$

n = Number of observations in the sample

11. Standard deviation from grouped data

For a population:

$$\sigma = \sqrt{\frac{\sum f(x - \mu)^2}{N}}$$

For a sample:

$$s = \sqrt{\frac{\sum f(x - \bar{x})^2}{n - 1}}$$

where

f = Absolute class frequencies
x = Class midpoints of grouped population (or sample) values
μ = Population
$\bar{x}$ = Sample
N = Number of observations in the population
n = Number of observations in the sample

12. Variance from ungrouped data—shortcut method

For a population:

$$\sigma^2 = \frac{\sum x^2 - N\mu^2}{N}$$

For a sample:

$$s^2 = \frac{\sum x^2 - n\bar{x}^2}{n - 1}$$

where

$\sum x^2$ = Sum of squared population (or sample) values
μ^2 = Squared population mean
$\bar{x}^2$ = Squared sample mean
N = Number of observations in the population
n = Number of observations in the sample

13. Variance from grouped data—shortcut method

For a population:

$$\sigma^2 = \frac{\sum fx^2 - N\mu^2}{N}$$

For a sample:

$$s^2 = \frac{\sum fx^2 - n\bar{x}^2}{n-1}$$

where

$\sum fX^2$ = Sum of absolute class frequency (f) times squared class midpoint (x) products

μ^2 = Squared population mean

$\bar{x}^2$ = Squared sample mean

N = Number of observations in the population

n = number of observations in the sample

II. FORMULAS FOR CALCULATING CONTROL CHART LIMITS

1. Control chart limits
   a. X-bar and R chart
   Process average

$$\text{UCL} = \bar{\bar{X}} + A_2\bar{R}$$

$$\text{Centerline} = \bar{\bar{X}}$$

$$\text{LCL} = \bar{\bar{X}} - A_2\bar{R}$$

Process variation

$$\text{UCL} = D_4\bar{R}$$

$$\text{Centerline} = \bar{R}$$

$$\text{LCL} = D_3\bar{R}$$

where

$$\text{UPC} = \text{Upper control limit of the process}$$

$$\text{LCL} = \text{Lower control limit of the process}$$

$$A_2, D_4, \text{ and } D_3 = \text{Constants}$$

$$\bar{\bar{X}} = \text{Process average}$$

$$\bar{R} = \text{Average range}$$

b. Individual (X) and moving range chart
Process average

$$\text{UCL} = \bar{\bar{X}} + E_2\bar{R}$$

Note that in this case the $\bar{X}$ and $\bar{\bar{X}}$ are the same.

$$\text{Centerline} = \bar{\bar{X}}$$

$$\text{LCL} = \bar{\bar{X}} - E_2\bar{R}$$

Process variation

$$\text{UCL} = D_4\bar{R}$$

$$\text{Centerline} = \bar{R}$$

$$\text{LCL} = D_3\bar{R}$$

where

$$\begin{aligned}
\text{UPC} &= \text{Upper control limit of the process}\\
\text{LCL} &= \text{Lower control limit of the process}\\
E_2, D_4, \text{ and } D_3 &= \text{Constants}\\
\bar{\bar{X}} &= \text{Process average}\\
\bar{R} &= \text{Average range}
\end{aligned}$$

To calculate the range, the experimenter must couple the individual data points in groups. The most sensitive (and recommended) grouping is a sample of two observations. More may be grouped together; however, much of the sensitivity will be lost.

c. X-bar and s chart
Process average

$$\text{UCL} = \bar{\bar{X}} + A_3\bar{s}$$

$$\text{Centerline} = \bar{\bar{X}}$$

$$\text{LCL} = \bar{\bar{X}} - A_3\bar{s}$$

Process variation

$$\text{UCL} = B_4\bar{s}$$

$$\text{Centerline} = \bar{s}$$

$$\text{LCL} = B_3\bar{s}$$

where

$$UPC = \text{Upper control limit of the process}$$
$$LCL = \text{Lower control limit of the process}$$
$$A_3, B_4, \text{ and } B_3 = \text{Constants}$$
$$\overline{\overline{X}} = \text{Process average}$$
$$\overline{s} = \text{Average standard deviation}$$

   d. Median chart
   Process average

$$UCL = \overline{\overline{X}} + \widetilde{A}_2 \overline{R}$$

$$\text{Centerline} = \overline{\overline{X}}$$

$$LCL = \overline{\overline{X}} - \widetilde{A}_2 \overline{R}$$

   Process variation

$$UCL = D_4 \overline{R}$$

$$\text{Centerline} = \overline{R}$$

$$LCL = D_3 \overline{R}$$

where

$$UPC = \text{Upper control limit of the process}$$
$$LCL = \text{Lower control limit of the process}$$
$$\widetilde{A}_2, D_4, \text{ and } D_3 = \text{Constants}$$
$$\overline{\overline{X}} = \text{Process median (median of all the sample medians)}$$
$$\overline{R} = \text{Average range}$$

   e. p-chart

$$UCL = \overline{p} + 3\sqrt{\frac{\overline{p}(1 - \overline{p})}{n}}$$

$$\text{Centerline} = \overline{p}$$

$$LCL = \overline{p} - 3\sqrt{\frac{\overline{p}(1 - \overline{p})}{n}}$$

where

UCL = Upper control limit of the process
LCL = Lower control limit of the process
$\bar{p}$ = Average proportion defective

f. np-chart

$$UCL = n\bar{p} + 3\sqrt{\frac{n\bar{p}(1-\bar{p})}{n}}$$

Centerline = $\bar{p}$

$$LCL = n\bar{p} - 3\sqrt{\frac{n\bar{p}(1-\bar{p})}{n}}$$

where

UCL = Upper control limit of the process
LCL = Lower control limit of the process
$n\bar{p}$ = Number of average proportion defective

g. Standardized-value p-chart

$$p_s = \frac{(p-\bar{p})}{\sqrt{\frac{\bar{p}\bar{q}}{n}}}$$

where

p_s = Standard p-value
p = Observed sample proportion defective
q = (1-p) yield
n = Sample size
$\bar{p}$ = Process average proportion defective

h. c-chart

$$UCL = \bar{c} + 3\sqrt{\bar{c}}$$

Centerline = $\bar{c}$

$$LCL = \bar{c} - 3\sqrt{\bar{c}}$$

where

UCL = Upper control limit of the process
LCL = Lower control limit of the process
$\bar{c}$ = average defect

i. u-chart

$$UCL = \bar{u} + 3\sqrt{\frac{\bar{u}}{n}}$$

Centerline = $\bar{u}$

$$LCL = \bar{u} - 3\sqrt{\frac{\bar{u}}{n}}$$

where

UCL = Upper control limit of the process
LCL = Lower control limit of the process
$\bar{u}$ = Average of the number defects

2. Capability
   a. Process capability

$$C_p = \frac{USL - LSL}{6\sigma_x}$$

where

USL = Upper specifications
LSL = Lower specifications
σ_x = Standard deviation

b. Capability ratio

$$C_r = \frac{6\sigma_x}{USL - LSL}$$

where

USL = Upper specifications
LSL = Lower specifications
σ_x = Standard deviation

c. Capability index

$$C_{pk} = \frac{Z_{min}}{3}$$

where

Z_{min} = Less value of (USL-Xbar)/3σ and (Xbar-LSL)/3σ

d. Target ratio percent

$$TR_p = \frac{3\sigma}{Z_{min}} \times 100$$

III. CONSTANTS IN CONTROL CHARTS

Sample Size (n)	Estimating sx			X Chart:		Median Chart:	Individual X Chart:	R Chart		s Chart	
	d-2	d-3	c-4	A-2	A-3	A-2	E-2	D-3	D-4	B-3	B-4
2	1.128	0.853	0.7979	1.880	2.659	1.880	2.660	0.000	3.267	0.000	3.267
3	1.693	0.888	0.8862	1.023	1.954	1.187	1.772	0.000	2.574	0.000	2.568
4	2.059	0.880	0.9213	0.729	1.628	0.796	1.457	0.000	2.282	0.000	2.266
5	2.326	0.864	0.9400	0.577	1.427	0.691	1.190	0.000	2.114	0.000	2.089
6	2.534	0.848	0.9515	0.483	1.287	0.548	1.184	0.000	2.004	0.030	1.970
7	2.704	0.833	0.9594	0.419	1.182	0.508	1.109	0.076	1.924	0.118	1.882
8	2.847	0.820	0.9650	0.373	1.099	0.433	1.054	0.136	1.864	0.185	1.815
9	2.970	0.808	0.9693	0.337	1.032	0.412	1.010	0.184	1.816	0.239	1.761
10	3.078	0.797	0.9727	0.308	0.975	0.362	0.975	0.223	1.777	0.284	1.761

Control Charts

This appendix provides the reader with some selected common control charts used in healthcare.

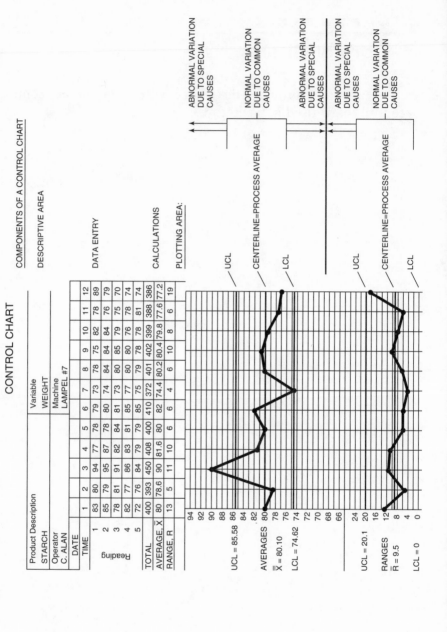

F I G U R E   G–2

Same X-bar and R Control Charts Using Computer Software

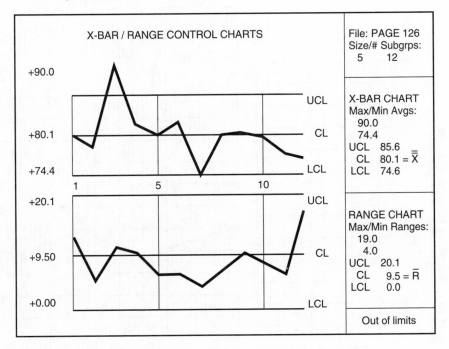

SgNo.	Data					Average	Range
1.	83	85	78	82	72	80.0	13
2.	80	79	81	77	76	78.6	5
3.	94	95	91	86	84	90.0	11
4.	77	87	82	83	79	81.6	10
5.	78	78	84	81	79	80.0	6
6.	79	80	81	85	85	82.0	6
7.	73	74	73	77	75	74.4	4
8.	78	84	80	80	79	80.2	6
9.	75	84	85	80	78	80.4	10
10.	82	84	79	76	78	79.8	8
11.	78	76	75	78	81	77.6	6
12.	89	79	70	74	74	77.2	19

FIGURE G-3   Typical Individual and Moving Range Charts

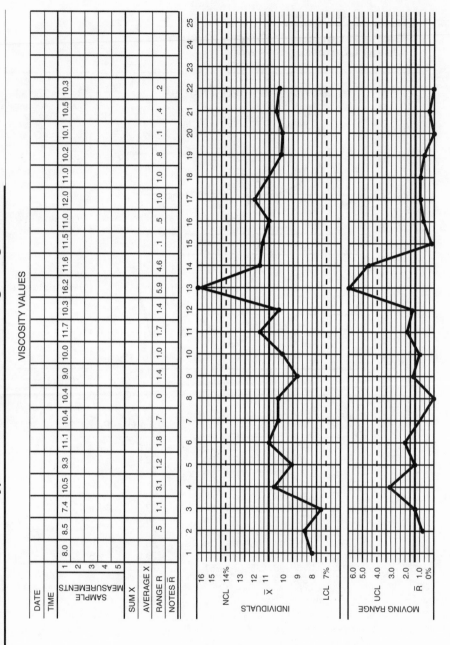

F I G U R E   G–4

Same Individual and Moving Range Control Charts Using Computer Software

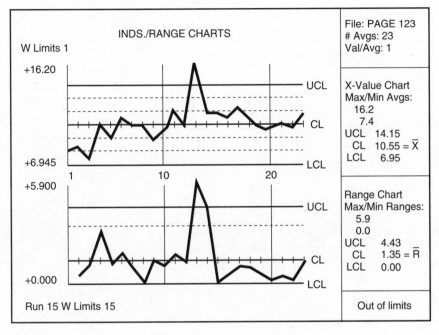

SgNo.	Data	Average	Range
1.	8.0	8.00	0.5
2.	8.5	8.50	0.5
3.	7.4	7.40	1.1
4.	10.5	10.50	3.1
5.	9.3	9.30	1.2
6.	11.1	11.10	1.8
7.	10.4	10.40	0.7
8.	10.4	10.40	0.0
9.	9.0	9.00	1.4
10.	10.0	10.00	1.0
11.	11.7	11.70	1.7
12.	10.3	10.30	1.4
13.	16.2	16.20	5.9
14.	11.6	11.60	4.6
15.	11.5	11.50	0.1
16.	11.0	11.00	0.5
17.	12.0	12.00	1.0
18.	11.0	11.00	1.0
19.	10.2	10.20	0.8
20.	10.1	10.10	0.1
21.	10.5	10.50	0.4
22.	10.3	10.30	0.2
23.	11.6	11.60	1.3

F I G U R E   G–5

Typical p-Chart

CONTROL CHART FOR ATTRIBUTE DATA

p ☑   c ☐
np ☐   w ☐

PART NUMBER AND NAME

DEPARTMENT — Lab

OPERATION NUMBER AND NAME — REBLENDING

PRODUCT ENGINEERING
DESIGNATED CONTROL ITEM (∇) ☐

Avg. = 5.83   UCL = .0769   LCL = .0397

Average Sample Size:
Frequency:

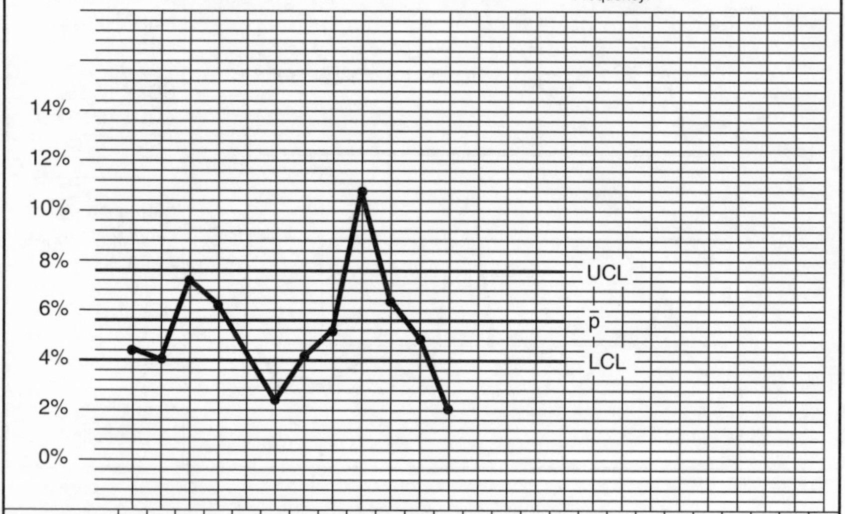

Sample (n)	1524	1275	1821	1496	1213	1371	1248	1123	1517	1488	2052	1696													
Number (np.c)	70	53	32	91	32	55	69	67	159	94	105	37													
Proportion (p.u.)	4.59	4.16	7.25	6.08	2.64	4.01	5.53	5.97	10.48	6.32	5.12	2.18													
Date	8/11	8/12	8/13	8/14	8/15	8/16	8/17	8/18	8/19	8/20	8/21	8/22													

(left margin label: Discrepancies)

ANY CHANGE IN PEOPLE, MATERIALS, EQUIPMENT, METHODS OR ENVIROMENT SHOULD BE NOTED.
THESE NOTES WILL HELP YOU TO TAKE CORRECTIVE OR PROCESS IMPROVEMENT ACTION WHEN
SIGNALED BY THE CONTROL CHART.

DATE	TIME	COMMENTS

(Over)

F I G U R E   G–6

Same p-Chart Using Computer Software

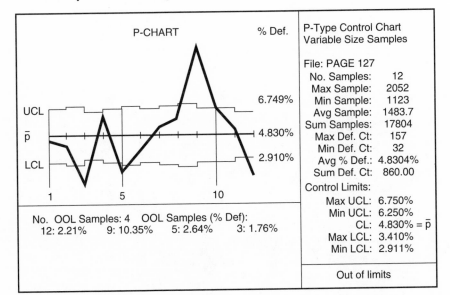

CtNo.	Count	Samp Sz	%Defective	U.C.L.%	L.C.L.%	Comment
1.	70	1524	4.593%	6.478%	3.183%	1. 8/11/87
2.	53	1275	4.157%	6.632%	3.029%	2. 8/12/87
3.	32	1821	1.757%	6.338%	3.323%	3. 8/13/87
4.	91	1496	6.083%	6.493%	3.167%	4. 8/14/87
5.	32	1213	2.638%	6.677%	2.984%	5. 8/15/87
6.	55	1371	4.012%	6.568%	3.093%	6. 8/16/87
7.	67	1248	5.369%	6.651%	3.010%	7. 8/17/87
8.	67	1123	5.966%	6.750%	2.911%	8. 8/18/87
9.	157	1517	10.349%	6.482%	3.179%	9. 8/19/87
10.	94	1488	6.317%	6.498%	3.163%	10. 8/20/87
11.	105	2052	5.117%	6.250%	3.410%	11. 8/21/87
12.	37	1676	2.208%	6.402%	3.259%	12. 8/22/87

This glossary provides some of the terms frequently used in the implementation of total quality management in healthcare.

Affinity chart   The organized output from a team brainstorming session, which uses cards as headers that can be changed and organized in piles for discussion.

Benefit   See outcome.

Boundary   The beginning or end point in the portion of a process from a supplier to a customer that will be the focus of the process improvement effort.

Brainstorming   A group decision-making technique designed to generate a large number of creative ideas through an interactive process. Brainstorming is used to generate alternative ideas to be considered in making decisions.

Capability   Can be determined only after the process is in statistical control. When the process average ± 3-sigma spread of the distribution of individuals is contained within the specification tolerance (variables data) or when at least 99.73 percent of individuals are within specification (attribute data), a process is said to be capable. Efforts to improve capability must continue consistent with the operational philosophy of never-ending improvement in quality and productivity.

Cause-and-effect chart   A graphic tool used to explore and display options about those components of a process that affect every occurrence. A cause-and-effect chart is used to clearly illustrate the various causes affecting a given key quality characteristic (KQC) by sorting and relating the causes to the effect as well as to create a starting point for determining the key process variables (KPV). It is also called the Fishbone diagram or Ishikawa diagram.

Center line   The line on a control chart that represents the average (mean or median) value of the items being plotted.

Check sheet   A data collection form consisting of multiple categories. Each category has an operational definition and can be checked off as it occurs. Properly designed, the check sheet helps to summarize the data, which are often displayed in a Pareto chart.

Coach   A key resource person from within the hospital who will support the CEO's leadership of the quality improvement process. A coach is a respected peer from the hospital workforce who is enthusiastic and knowledgeable about quality improvement and eager both to learn and to help others learn.

Common-cause variation   The inherent variation of the process. It is the result of interactions within the process that affect every occurrence. See also process variation.

Control chart   A display of data in the order that they occur with statistically determined upper and lower limits of expected common cause variation. It is used to indicate special causes of process variation, to monitor a process for maintenance, and to determine if process changes have had the desired effect.

Control limits   Expected limits of common cause variation. Sometimes they are referred to as upper and lower control limits. They are not specification or tolerance limits.

Correlation chart   A chart that shows the relationship between two variables.

Cross-functional team   See team.

Customer   The receiver of an output of a process, either internal or external to a hospital or corporate unit. A customer could be a person, a department, a company, and so on. In healthcare it is certainly more than the patient.

Data collection   Gathering facts on how a process works and/or how a process is working from the customer's point of view. All data collection is driven by knowledge of the process and is guided by statistical principles.

Deming cycle for continuous improvement   A visualization of the quality improvement process usually consisting of four points—Plan, Do, Check (Study), Act—linked by quarter circles. The cycle was first developed by Dr. W. A. Shewhart but was popularized in Japan in the 1950s by Dr. W. E. Deming.

Deming's 14 principles   The foundation on which the organizationwide quality improvement process is built. The points are a blend of leadership, management theory, and statistical concepts, which highlight the responsibilities of management while enhancing the capacities of employees.

Distribution diagram   A diagram that shows the frequencies of the variables in a predetermined grouping.

Fishbone diagram   See cause-and-effect chart.

Flowchart   A graphic representation of the flow of a process. A flowchart is a useful way to examine how various steps in a process relate to each other; define the boundaries of the process; identify customer–supplier relationships in a process; verify or form the appropriate team; create a common understanding of the process flow; determine the current best method of performing the process; and identify redundancy, unnecessary complexity, and inefficiency in a process.

FOCUS-PDCA   A strategy that provides a road map for continuous process improvement when linked to a quality definition. The acronym means: Find a process to improve, Organize a team that knows the process, Clarify the current knowledge of the process, Understand causes of process variation, Select the process improvement, Plan the improvement and continued data collection, Do the improvement (data collection and analysis), Check and study the results, *Act* to hold the gain and to continue to improve the process.

Force field analysis (FFA)   A systematic method for understanding competing forces that increase or decrease the likelihood of successfully implementing change. It provides a framework for developing change strategies aimed at decreasing restraining forces and increasing driving forces.

Functional team   A group of five to eight people addressing an issue in which any recommended changes would not be likely to affect people outside the specific area. For example, a functional team concerned with filing and retrieving data in the laboratory might consist just of people who work in the lab.

Future state   A description of an organization that has gone through a quality improvement process transformation. In this state, explicit messages from the leadership clearly and consistently support and reinforce the new way. People work more efficiently together. Common language evolves related to mission, customers, and daily organizational life. Standards are never enough, and the status quo is never good enough. Listening to customers is the driving philosophy of the organization.

Hospital quality trends (HQT)   A series of reports used in many hospitals on judgments of key customers about hospital quality, such as patients—a report on patient judgments. HQT is a systematic method of listening to the voice of the customer for the continuous improvement of quality.

Ishikawa diagram   See cause-and-effect diagram.

Key process variable (KPV)   A component of the process that has a cause-and-effect relationship of sufficient magnitude with the key quality characteristic (KQC), such that manipulation and control of the KPV will reduce variation of the KQC and/or change its level.

Key quality characteristic (KQC)   The most important quality characteristic. KQC must be operationally defined by combining knowledge of the customer with knowledge of the process.

Matrix chart   A format that is used in deploying quality requirements into counterpart specific characteristics and then into product/service requirements.

Matrix data analysis   This diagram is used when the matrix chart does not provide sufficient detailed information.

Mentor   A highly skilled quality improvement process (QIP) professional with extensive training and experience in the initiation and operation of an organizationwide quality improvement process. A mentor is an external resource person who visits periodically to counsel the CEO and other leaders in the initiation of the improvement process.

Multidisciplinary team   See team.

Multiple voting   A group decision-making technique designed to reduce a long list to a few ideas.

New quality technology tools   A group of techniques and charts used to collect, organize, display, and evaluate knowledge about a process. Specifically, they are affinity chart, correlation chart, distribution diagram, matrix chart, matrix data analysis, process decision program chart (PDPC), and program evaluation review technique (PERT).

Old quality tools   A group of techniques and charts used to collect, organize, display, and evaluate knowledge about a process. Specifically, they are brainstorming, flow chart, cause-and-effect chart, check sheet, Pareto chart, histogram, run chart, and control chart.

Operational definition   A description in quantifiable terms of what to measure and the steps to follow to consistently measure it. The purpose of this measurement is to determine the actual performance of the process. An operational definition is developed for each key quality characteristic before data are collected.

Opportunity statement   A concise description of a process in need of improvement, its boundaries, and the general area of concern where a quality improvement team should begin its efforts.

Outcome (benefit)   The degree to which outputs meet the needs and expectations of the customer.

Output   What is produced by the actions of the process.

Owner   The person who has or is given the responsibility and authority to lead the continuing improvement of a process. Process ownership is driven by the boundaries of the process.

Paradigm shift   A point in time when the knowledge or structure that underlies a science or discipline changes in such a fundamental way that the beliefs and behavior of the people involved in the science or discipline are changed. Many people feel a major paradigm shift is under way today in the healthcare field as the traditions of samaritan (helping) and science begin to include social accountability.

Pareto chart   A bar graph used to arrange information in such a way that priorities for process improvement can be established. It displays the relative impor-

---

* PDPC is an application of the process decision program chart used in operations research. This diagram was developed to optimize solutions and to avoid surprises.

* PERT. A chart designed to provide multiple pieces of information on a project. It is primarily used for very complex projects, although simple projects may benefit from its application.

tance of data and is used to direct efforts to the biggest improvement opportunity by highlighting the vital few in contrast to the many others.

Present state   A description of an organization as it currently exists. It includes what is happening now, both formally and informally in the organization—the status quo. In the present state, managers at all levels and employees throughout the organization are pulling in different directions because of diverse demands; short-term requirements; and unclear values, goals, and roles.

Process   A series of actions that repeatedly come together to transform inputs provided by a supplier into outputs received by a customer. All work is a process.

Process improvement   The continuous endeavor to learn about all aspects of a process and to use this knowledge to change the process to reduce variation and complexity and to improve customer judgments of quality. Process improvement begins by understanding how customers judge quality, how processes work, and how understanding the variation in those processes can lead to wise management action.

Process owner   See owner.

Process variation   The spread of process output over time. There is variation in every process, and all variation is caused. The causes are of two types: (1) normal, common, or inherent and (2) special or assignable. A process can have both types of variation at the same time or only the common-cause variation. The management action necessary to improve the process is very different in each situation.

Quality assurance   A term with two definitions. In traditional healthcare circles, it is the process established to meet external regulatory requirements, including those of the Joint Commission on Accreditation of Healthcare Organizations, and to assure that patient care is consistent with established standards. It also supports the medical staff credentialing procedures. In modern quality terms, quality assurance means designing a product or service so well that quality is inevitable.

Quality characteristics   Characteristics of the output of a process that are important to the customer. The identification of quality characteristics requires knowledge of the customer needs and expectations.

Quality control   A traditional, outdated way of thinking about quality. The focus of quality control is always on appraising systems after the product or service has been delivered. It is a sorting mechanism.

Quality improvement council (QIC)   A group composed of the coach and a senior leader of an organization, which is primarily responsible for planning, strategy development, deployment, monitoring, educating, and promoting the quality improvement process.

Quality improvement process (QIP)   The application of new quality technology tools in the day-to day operation and management of an organization. The insights of Drs. W. Edwards Deming, Joseph M. Juran, and Kaoru Ishikawa as well as Professor Shigeru Mizuno and many others form the basis for this transformation.

Quality improvement storytelling   A major accelerator of the process of organizationwide quality improvement that uses quality improvement storybooks to follow steps in the FOCUS-PDCA strategy. Storybooks and storyboards help teams organize their work and their presentations so that others can more readily learn from them. Use of storyboards and storybooks reduces variation in the process of quality improvement storytelling so the focus of learning is on content, not the method of telling. Storybooks form a permanent record of a team's actions and achievements and all the data generated, and storyboards can function as the working minutes of a team.

Quality improvement team (QIT)   A specially constituted group, usually five to eight people, chosen to address a specific opportunity for improvement. This team consists of people who have regular contact with the process.

Quality inspection   Usually consists of three stages: sampling, measuring, and sorting. Although many organizations rely on inspection to improve quality, the better way is to design quality into the product or service, to improve the process. This may include some inspection as a means of data gathering.

Quality management process (QMP)   Same as quality improvement process.

Quality tools   See new and old quality technology tools.

Red bead experiment   A simple exercise to demonstrate, among other things, that many managers hold workers to standards beyond their control, variation is part of any process, and workers work within a system beyond their control. The game also shows that some workers will always be above average, some average, and some below average; that the system, not the skills of individual workers, determines to a large extent how workers in repeating processes perform; and that only management can change the system or empower others to change it.

Refreezing   Recognizing, reinforcing, and rewarding new organizational attitudes and behaviors so they become the norm. Refreezing involves making processes, systems, and methods throughout the organization support the quality improvement process.

Rework   The act of doing something again because it was not done right the first time. It can occur for a variety of reasons, including insufficient planning, failure of a customer to specify the needed input, and failure of a supplier to provide a consistently high quality output.

Run   A point or a consecutive number of points that are above or below the central line in a run chart. Too long a run or too many or two few runs can be evidence of the existence of special causes of variation.

Run chart   A display of data in the order that they occur. A run chart is used to indicate the presence of special causes of process variation in the form of trends, shifts, or other nonrandom patterns in a key quality characteristic.

Shewhart cycle   See Deming cycle for continuous improvement.

Special cause variation   Variation in the process that does not affect every occurrence but arises because of special circumstances.

Sponsor   The person or group of people responsible for making the business decision that improving the process is important enough to provide team members and a coach or facilitator adequate time and resources to work on the improvement. The sponsor is most often a department manager or the quality improvement council.

Statistical thinking for process improvement   A data-driven method for decision making based primarily on an understanding of process variation. It results in wise management actions that contribute to the continuous improvement of quality.

Storyboard   See quality improvement storytelling.

Storybook   See quality improvement storytelling.

Storytelling   See quality improvement storytelling.

Supplier   The party or entity responsible for an input to a process. A supplier could be a person, department, a company, and so on. A supplier differs from a vendor in that the supplier relationship is always win-win. A vendor relationship is that of a commodity or price and therefore win-lose.

Tampering   Taking action without taking into account the difference between special and common-cause variation.

Team leader   A person designated to lead the quality improvement team who has team leadership skills and basic quality improvement skills.

Team (cross-functional and multidisciplinary)   A group of usually five to nine people from two or more areas of an organization who are addressing an issue that has an impact on the operations of each area. For example, the processes of distributing laboratory results might be addressed by a team involving laboratory, nursing, and medical staff. See also functional team.

Tools   See new and old quality technology tools.

Transformation   A major organizational change from the present state to a new and preferred state in which the quality improvement process flourishes. The primary steps involved in moving an organization through a transformation are present state, unfreezing, transition period, refreezing, and new/preferred state.

Transition period   A description of the time when an organization is visibly moving away from the old way toward the new way. During this time, employee attitudes and behaviors range from being excited and busy to being confused and resistant. The support for change builds. New leaders emerge, champions of the change come forward, and confusion over roles begins to clear.

Unfreezing   Reassessing old values and behaviors and becoming open to the acceptance of a new culture.

Variation   See process variation.

Vendor   See supplier.

BIBLIOGRAPHY

Advisory Board Company. *TQM: 14 Tactics for Improving the Quality Process*. Advisory Board Company, 1992.

Al-Assaf, A. F., and J. A. Schmele, eds. *Total Quality in Health Care*. Delray Beach, Fla.: St. Lucie Press, 1994.

Aloian, D. C., and W. R. Fowler. "How to Create a High Performance Training Plan." *Training and Development*, November 1994, pp. 43–44.

Atchison, T. "TQM the Questionable Movement?" *Healthcare Financial Management* 46, no. 3 (1992), pp. 15, 19.

Avolio, B. J. "The Alliance of Total Quality and the Full Range of Leadership." In B. M. Bass and B. J. Avolio, eds. *Improving Organizational Effectiveness through Transformational Leadership*. Thousand Oaks, Calif.: Sage, 1993.

Baker, E. M., and H. L. Artinian. "The Deming Philosophy of Continuing Improvement in a Service Organization. *Quality Progress*, June 1985, pp. 61–69.

Bass, M. "Creating a Climate for Change." *American Journal of Nursing*, March 1993 (Supplement), pp. 11–15.

Bass, B. M. *Leadership and Performance beyond Expectations*. New York: Free Press, 1985.

Batchelor, C. J., and T. H. Esmond, Jr. "Maintaining High Quality Patient Care while Controlling Costs." *Healthcare Financial Management* 43, no. 2 (1989), pp. 20–30.

Berger, S. "Quality Assessment Strategy Should Be Applied Consistently." *Modern Healthcare*, May 30, 1994, p. 34.

Berwick, D. M. "Continuous Improvement as an Ideal in Health Care." *New England Journal of Medicine* 320 (November 1989), pp. 53–57.

Best, K. "Conquering the TQM Learning Curve." *Contemporary Long Term Care* 16, no. 10 (1993), pp. 40–42, 44, 94.

Bhote, K. R. *World-Class Quality: Using Design of Experiments to Make It Happen*. Milwaukee: Quality Press, 1991.

Blackwell, G. "The New Frontier of Multimedia." *Canadian Business,* November 1991, pp. 85–94.

Boyd, M. "Motivating on a Dime." *Performance,* March 1995, pp. 62–65.

Bragar, J. "The Customer-Focused Quality Leader." *Quality Progress,* May 1992, pp. 51–53.

Brewer, G. "The New Manager." *Performance,* March 1995, pp. 30–35.

———. "The Goldfus Rule." *Successful Meetings,* June 1995, pp. 18–23.

Burney, R. "TQM in a Surgery Center." *Quality Progress,* January 1994, pp. 97–100.

Byrne, J. "The Horizontal Corporation." *Business Week,* December 20, 1993, pp. 76–81.

Califano, J. A., Jr. "Billions Wasted: At Least a Fourth of American Health Care Dollars Are Misspent." *New York Times,* April 16, 1989, p. 10.

Clark, S. "Quality Isn't Enough; Programs Need to Be Market Driven." *Marketing News,* June 10, 1991, p. 15.

Clarke, P., and D. Murray. "Information Technology in Customer Service." *Business Quarterly,* Spring 1990, pp. 91–94.

Clement, J. P. "Vertical Integration and Diversification of Acute Care Hospitals: Conceptual Definitions." *Hospital and Health Services Administration* 33, no. 5 (1988), pp. 99–110.

Cole, R. E. "Organizational Obstacles to Quality Improvement or: 'Beyond SPC.' " *Liaison Office Newsletter,* Fall 1987, p. 3–4.

Coleman, G. D., and E. M. Van Aken. "Applying Small-Group Behavior Dynamics to Improve Action-Team Performance." *Employment Relations Today,* Autumn 1991, pp. 343–53.

Coleman, L. G. "Total Quality Management Prescribed as Cure for Healthcare Ailments." *Marketing News,* May 11, 1992, pp. 5, 8.

Collier, D. A. "The Customer Service and Quality Challenge." *Service Industries Journal,* January 1987, pp. 77–90.

Conger, J. "Inspiring Others: The Language of Leadership. *Academy of Management Executives,* February 1991, pp. 31–45.

Crosby, P. B. *Quality Is Free.* New York: McGraw-Hill, 1979.

Dallaire, R. M. "Data-Based Marketing for Competitive Advantage." *Information Strategy,* Spring 1992, pp. 5–9.

Davis, V. "Self Audits, First Step in TQM." *HR Magazine* 37, no. 9 (1992), pp. 39–41.

Deming, W. E. *Out of the Crisis.* Cambridge, Mass.: MIT Center for Advanced Engineering Study, 1986.

———. "Drastic Changes for Western Management." Paper presented. *Proceedings of TIMS/ORS,* Gold Coast City, Australia, July 15–18, 1986.

———. "Need for Change." Letter distributed at seminar at Ford's world headquarters, Dearborn, Mich., March 1988.

———. "Some Notes on a Stable Process, and on Tampering." Letter distributed at seminar at Ford's world headquarters, Dearborn, Mich., October 1988.

———. "Foundation for Management of Quality in the Western World." rev. ed. Paper presented at Institute of Management Sciences, Osaka, Japan, April 1, 1990.

Denton, D. K. "Building a Team." *Quality Progress,* October 1992, pp. 87–91.

Donabedian, A. *The Definition of Quality and Approaches to Its Assessment.* Ann Arbor, Mich.: Health Administration Press, 1980.

Donoho, R. "Conflict and Carter." *Successful Meetings,* June 1995, pp. 38–45.

Dusharme, D. "The Real World according to TQM." *Quality Digest,* September 1994, pp. 34–39.

Emery, J. C. "Information Technology in the 21st Century Enterprise." *MIS Quarterly,* December 1991, pp. xxi–xxiii.

Feigenbaum, A. "TQM: Healthcare Can Learn from Other Fields." *Hospitals* 66, no. 22 (1992), p. 56.

Finison, L. J. "What Are Good Health Care Measurements?" *Quality Progress,* April 1992, pp. 41–44.

Frame, R. M., and W. R. Nielsen. "Excellence according to Plan." *Training and Development,* October 1988, pp. 37–39.

Furey, T. R. "How Information Power Can Improve Service Quality." *Planning Review,* May/June 1991, pp. 24–26.

Garvin, D. A. *Managing Quality.* New York: Free Press, 1988.

Giacalone, R. A., and P. Rosenfeld. *Impression Management in the Organization.* Hillsdale, N.J.: Lawrence Erlbaum, 1989.

Gillem, T. R. "Deming's 14 Points and Hospital Quality: Responding to the Consumer's Demand for the Best Value Health Care." *Journal of Nursing Quality Assurance* 2, no. 3 (1988), pp. 70–78.

Gillis, M. A. "Technology Alone Won't Bring Better Service." *ABA Banking Journal,* November 1989, p. 78.

Gottlier, M. "Hospital's Ethical Quandaries in Crunch to Pass Inspection." *New York Times,* March 12, 1992, pp. A1, B4.

Hall, R. A. "Technology: The Key to Customer Service during the 1990s." *Pension World,* March 1992, pp. 14–15.

Hart, C. W. L., and C. E. Bogan. *The Baldrige.* New York: McGraw-Hill, 1992.

Hauser, J. R., and D. Clausing. "The House of Quality." *Harvard Business Review,* May–June 1988, pp. 63–73.

Herzlinger, R. E. "The Failed Revolution in Healthcare: The Role of Management." *Harvard Business Review,* March–April 1989, pp. 95–103.

Hewitt, S. "Strategic Advantages Emerge from Tactical TQM Tools." *Quality Progress,* October 1994, pp. 57–60.

Hoexter, R., and M. Julien. "Legal Eagles Become Quality Hawks." *Quality Progress,* January 1994, pp. 31–34.

"Hospitals/Service Master Survey Tracks TQM/CQI." *Hospitals,* June 20, 1992, p. 44.

House, R. J. "A Theory of Charismatic Leadership." In J. G. Hunt and L. L. Larson, eds. *Leadership: The Cutting Edge.* Carbondale, Ill.: Southern Illinois University Press, 1977.

Hurt, F. "Better Brainstorming." *Training and Development,* November 1994, pp. 57–59.

Hutchinson, D. *Total Quality Management in the Clinical Laboratory.* Milwaukee: Quality Press, 1994.

———. "Chaos Theory, Complexity Theory, and Health Care Quality Management." *Quality Progress,* November 1994, pp. 69–72.

Isgar, T.; J. Ranney; and S. Grinnell. "Team Leaders: The Key to Quality." *Training and Development,* April 1994, pp. 45–47.

Ishikawa, K. *What Is Quality Control? The Japanese Way.* New York: Free Press, 1985.

Jacobs, P. "EDI, Imaging Exploding." *Computerworld,* January 20, 1992, p. 80.

Jessup, P. T. "The Value of Continuing Improvement." In *Proceedings of the International Communications Conference.* Boston, Mass: International Communications Conference, 1985.

Juran, J. M. *Juran on Planning for Quality.* New York: Free Press, 1988.

———. *Juran in Leadership for Quality.* New York: Free Press, 1989.

———. "The Upcoming Century of Quality." *Quality Progress,* August 1994, pp. 29–38.

Kaluzny, A. "Managing Transitions: Assuring the Adaptation and Impact of TQM." *Quality Review Bulletin* 18, no. 11 (1992), pp. 380–84.

King, B. *Better Designs in Half the Time: Implementing QFD in America.* Methuen, Mass.: GOAL/QPC, 1987.

Knouse, S. B. *The Reward and Recognition Process in Total Quality Management.* Milwaukee: Quality Press, 1995.

Kobayashi, I. *20 Keys to Work Place Improvement.* Cambridge, Mass.: Productivity Press, 1990.

Kongstvedt, P. R. *Essentials of Managed Health Care.* Frederick, Md.: Aspen Publishers, 1995.

Kouzes, J., and B. Posner. *The Leadership Challenge.* San Francisco: Jossey Bass, 1995.

Kovner, M. A. "Outcomes Assessment Using Medis Groups: A Case Study." Presented at the National Healthcare Quality Conference, Louisville, Ky., September 17–18, 1990.

Krulikowski, C. "Measuring Employee Satisfaction." *Quality Digest,* September 1994, pp. 58–65.

Kuhnert, K. W. "Transforming Leadership." In B. M. Bass and B. J. Avolio, eds. *Improving Organizational Effectiveness through Transformational Leadership.* Thousand Oaks, Calif.: Sage, 1993.

Laffel, G. "Implementing Quality Management in Healthcare: The Challenges Ahead." *Quality Progress,* November 1990, pp. 29–32.

Laffel, G., and D. Blumenthal. "The Case for Using Industrial Quality Management Science in Health Care Organizations." *Journal of the American Medical Association* 262 (1989), pp. 2869–73.

Lahiry, S. "Building Commitment through Organizational Culture." *Training and Development,* April 1994, pp. 50–52.

Landrum, R. "12 Reasons to Implement ISO 9000." *Quality Digest,* December 1993, pp. 39–42.

Lee, C. "Beyond Teamwork." *Training,* June 1990, pp. 25–32.

Leedy, K., and J. Lloyd. "Malcolm Baldrige National Quality Award and the Healthcare Forum/Witt Commitment to Quality Award." Presented at the National Healthcare Quality Conference, Louisville, Ky., September 17–18, 1990.

Lumphhrey, D. "TQM to the Rescue." *Medical Laboratory Observer* 25, no. 5 (1993), pp. 33–36, 38.

Lutz, S. "Not-for-Profits Up for Grabs by the Giants." *Modern Healthcare*, May 30, 1994, pp. 24–28.

Lutz, S. "NME to Pay Fine of $379 Million." *Modern Healthcare*, July 4, 1994, pp. 2, 13.

MacStravic, S. "Scale Scoring in Health Care Customer Surveys." *Quirk's Marketing Research Review*, February 1994, pp. 12–15.

McDonell, E. D., and G. E. Somerville. "Corporate Reengineering That Follows the Design of Document Imaging." *Information Strategy*, Fall 1991, pp. 5–10.

McGrath, R. G. "Regaining Competitive Advantage through Leadership." *Quality Progress*, December 1993, pp. 109–12.

Merron, K. A. "Creating TQM Organizations." *Quality Progress*, January 1994, pp. 51–56.

Merry, M. "Illusion vs. Reality: TQM beyond the Yellow Brick Road." *Healthcare Executive* 6, no. 2 (1991), pp. 18–21.

Milakovich, M. "Total Quality Management for Public Service Productivity Improvement." *Public Productivity and Management Review* 14 (1991), pp. 19–32.

Milakovich, M. E. "Creating a Total Quality Health Care Environment." *Health Care Management Review* 16, no. 1 (1991), pp. 9–20.

Neches, P. M. "Major Technology Trends for the 1990s." *Financial Executive*, July/August 1991, pp. 11–15.

Newbold, P. A. "Quality through People: Memorial Health System's Approach to Quality Improvement." Presented at the National Healthcare Quality Conference, Louisville, Ky., September 17–18, 1990.

Niven, D. "When Times Get Tough, What Happens to TQM?" *Harvard Business Review* 71, no. 3 (1993), pp. 20–29.

Omachonu, V. K. "Quality of Care and the Patient: New Criteria for Evaluation." *Health Care Management Review*, Fall 1990, pp. 43–50.

O'Sullivan, D. D., and S. D. Grujic. "Implementing Hospital-Wide Quality Assurance." *Quality Progress*, February 1991, pp. 28–32.

Packer, A. "Preparing Work Force 2000." *Human Capital*, November–December 1993, pp. 34–38.

Pasternak, D. P., and J. A. Berry. "Health Care's Multiple Dimensions of Quality." *Quality Progress*, December 1993, pp. 87–96.

Pearce, T. *Leading Out Loud*. San Francisco: Jossey Bass, 1995.

Peters, T. *Thriving on Chaos: A Handbook for a Management Revolution*. New York: Alfred A. Knopf, 1987.

Powell, J. L. *Pathways to Leadership*. San Francisco: Jossey Bass, 1995.

Quinn, J. B., and P. C. Paquette. "Technology in Services: Creating Organizational Revolutions." *McKinsey Quarterly* 3 (1990), pp. 91–112.

Rankin, C., and K. T. Von Rueden. "Learning to Lead." *American Journal of Nursing*, March 1993 (Supplement), pp. 16–19.

Rozum, J. "A Way to Improve Customer Satisfaction." *Quality Progress*, October 1994, pp. 67–72.

Sheridan, B. M. "Changing Service Quality in America." *Quality Progress*, December 1993, pp. 97–100.

Scherkenback, W. W. *The Deming Route to Quality and Productivity.* Rockville, Md.: Mercury Press, 1986.

Schwarz, R. M. *The Skilled Facilitator.* San Francisco: Jossey Bass, 1994.

Showstack, J. A.; R. E. Rosenfeld; and D. W. Garnick. "Association of Volume with Outcome of Coronary Bypass Surgery: Scheduled vs. Nonscheduled Operations." *Journal of the American Medical Association* 257 (1987), pp. 785–89.

Shycon, H. N. "Improved Customer Service: Measuring the Payoff." *Journal of Business Strategy,* January/February 1992, pp. 13–17.

Simon, M. "Research with Health Care Providers: An Uncommon Approach to a Common Problem." *Quirk's Marketing Research Review,* June/July 1994, pp. 8–9, 28.

Simpson, R. L. "Benchmarking MIS Performance." *Nursing Management,* January 1994, pp. 20–21.

Sirkin, H., and G. Stalk, Jr. "Fix the Process not the Problem." *Harvard Business Review,* July–August 1990, pp. 26–33.

Slater, D. "IS at Your Service." *Computerworld,* January 20, 1992, pp. 71–73.

———. "Keeping Customers Happy Is Top Job for IS." *Computerworld,* December 23, 1991, pp. 2–3.

Slater, R. H. *Integrated Process Management: A Quality Model.* Milwaukee: Quality Press, 1991.

Snee, R. D. "Creating Robust Work Processes." *Quality Progress,* February 1993, pp. 37–41.

Starr, P. *The Social Transformation of American Medicine.* New York: Basic Books, 1982.

Stayer, R. "How I Learned to Let My Workers Lead." *Harvard Business Review,* November–December 1990, pp. 66–83.

Summers, L. "A Logical Approach to Development Planning." *Training and Development,* November 1994, pp. 22–31.

Szabo, J. C. "Service-Survival." *Nation's Business,* March 1989, pp. 16–24.

Tomasko, R. M. *Rethinking the Corporation: The Architecture of Change.* New York: AMACOM, 1993.

Townsend, P. L. *Commit to Quality.* New York: John Wiley & Sons, 1990.

Tuckman, B. W. "Developmental Sequence in Small Groups." *Psychological Bulletin* 63, no. 6 (1965), pp. 384–99.

Walbert, L. "Healthcare Reform: Reality Is at the Bedside." *CFO,* December 1993, pp. 22–26.

Walton, M. *The Deming Management Method.* New York: Putnam, 1986.

———. "Deming's Parable of the Red Beads." *Across the Board,* February 1987, pp. 12–15.

Wellins, R. S.; W. C. Byham; and G. R. Dixon. *Inside Teams.* San Francisco: Jossey Bass, 1994.

Wennberg, J. E. "Which Rate Is Right?" *New England Journal of Medicine* 314 (1986), pp. 310–11.

Wurster, R. "Plans Don't Work—People Do." *Quality Progress,* March 1966, p. 5.

Yukl, G. *Leadership in Organizations.* 2d ed. New York: Academic Press, 1989.

Zablocki, E. *Changing Physician Practice Patterns.* Frederick, Md.: Aspen Publishers, 1995.

INDEX